Nature's Civil War

CIVIL WAR AMERICA

Gary W. Gallagher,

Peter S. Carmichael,

Caroline E. Janney,

and

Aaron Sheehan-Dean,

editors

Nature's
CIVIL WAR

Common Soldiers and the Environment

in 1862 Virginia

Kathryn Shively Meier

The University of North Carolina Press / Chapel Hill

This book was published with the assistance of the Fred W. Morrison Fund
for Southern Studies of the University of North Carolina Press.

The paper in this book meets the guidelines for permanence and durability
of the Committee on Production Guidelines for Book Longevity of the Council on
Library Resources. The University of North Carolina Press has been a member
of the Green Press Initiative since 2003.

Library of Congress Cataloging-in-Publication Data
Meier, Kathryn Shively.
Nature's Civil War : common soldiers and the environment in 1862 Virginia /
Kathryn Shively Meier.
pages cm. — (Civil War America)
Includes bibliographical references and index.
ISBN 978-1-4696-1076-4 (cloth : alk. paper)
1. United States—History—Civil War, 1861–1865—Health aspects—Virginia.
2. United States—History—Civil War, 1861–1865—Environmental aspects—Virginia.
3. Self-care, Health—Virginia—History—19th century. 4. Self-care, Health—United
States—History—19th century. 5. Military life—Virginia—History—19th century.
6. Military life—United States—History—19th century. I. Title. II. Title:
Common soldiers and the environment in 1862 Virginia.
E621.M45 2013
973.7′75—dc23
2013015620

Portions of this book were previously published in somewhat different form:
"'No Place for the Sick': Nature's War on Civil War Soldier Mental and Physical
Health in the 1862 Peninsula and Shenandoah Valley Campaigns," *Journal of the
Civil War Era* 1, no. 2 (2011); and "The Lost Boys," *Civil War Monitor* 2,
no. 3 (2012). Used with permission.

To
Louise, Jack, and Mark

Contents

Maps, Illustrations, Figures, and Tables

Acknowledgments

At one point in time, the manuscript of this book was absurdly replete with examples and unnecessarily didactic. Good-natured and highly respectable people more than did their parts in attempting to steer me back toward good history. All remaining folly is mine.

Chief among these people is Gary W. Gallagher. His advice kept me in graduate school in dark days, and his unflagging support and trust has bolstered my work and career incalculably since then. The passion and intellect he has dedicated to Civil War history make it impossible to imagine the field without him. I am profoundly grateful for his assistance on this project and astounded at my good fortune in being able to call him my mentor. Simply put, I would not be a historian if it weren't for Gary.

Other scholars at the University of Virginia groomed this project when it was a mere twinkle in my eye. Edward Ayers, one of the busier men alive, set aside hours to counsel me through considerable growing pains and to sharpen the ideas contained herein. He is an intellectual force of nature and a man of boundless generosity. Edmund Russell, a leader among environmental historians, introduced me to a subfield I now cherish, and he took special care to help train me as a professional. His humility and meticulous work continue to inspire me. In an early draft, Margaret Mohrmann gently corrected my medical errors with good humor (though by no means should remaining gaffes be associated with her).

Archives and the people who run them helped to form the backbone of this project, the research. I am thankful to the special collections staff at the University of Virginia and the Library of Virginia, both treasures of Civil War collections. A large portion of my research was completed at the Military History Institute of the U.S. Army War College, where Martin Andresen gave generously of his time, despite being retired, and Richard Sommers kindly thought to check up on me. At the Museum of the Confederacy, John Coski provides a munificent welcome to all scholars and extended his resources to me. Other institutions critically provided funding for my project. The Suzanne and Caleb Loring Civil War Fellowship, which I held jointly at the Massachusetts Historical Society and Boston Athenaeum, provided invaluable research as well as comfortable spaces to ponder and write. I am sincerely indebted to Conrad Wright and also Peter Drummey, Sara Georgini, and Jeremy Dibbell at the MHS and Mary Warnement and Stephen Nonack at the Athenaeum, who provided feedback, support, and opportunities for public lectures during my stay in Boston. A well-timed Gilder Lehrman fellowship allowed me to sift through the U.S. Sanitary Commission papers at the New York Public Library, thanks to the help of Thomas Lannon, completing my research.

Mark Simpson-Vos sought out this project when I was a very green historian and then cultivated it for many years. In the process, he has proven to be an exceptional editor. At critical moments, he offered sage advice and encouragement, which helped turn the corner in a sometimes grueling journey. David Perry has also given freely of his time, while the readers' reports helped to condense and refine the monograph, significantly enhancing its impacts. Series editor Peter Carmichael partook in the agony and, dare I say, the ecstasy of finally getting this manuscript off his desk. In between, he proved himself a perceptive and scrupulous editor, seeing value and complexity in my ideas of which I occasionally lost sight. Further, I am humbled and honored that this project was awarded the inaugural Edward M. Coffman First-Manuscript Prize by the Society for Military Historians in 2011. I delight in counting myself as one of the many young military scholars that Dr. Coffman has encouraged in his venerable career.

I consider many other readers of this project as esteemed colleagues and trusted friends. At the University of Scranton, David Dzurec has cheerfully shared with me the growing pains of developing a first manuscript. Professional opportunities brought me into contact with the infectiously ebullient Megan Kate Nelson, whose readings critically sharpened my prose and analysis, as well as the talented Aaron Sachs and his posse of discerning graduate students, who took me to task on chapter 5, and finally the munificent William Blair, whose character and scholarship inspires me. Bill is a tireless advocate of young scholars. Rachel Shelden has always championed my work, even when my own enthusiasm lagged. My career (let alone this book) would not have come to fruition without the editorial facility, wise counsel, and devoted friendship of Laura Kolar and Philip Mills Herrington. Peter Luebke is the most meticulous steward of Civil War scholarship imaginable. He has read this manuscript more times than anyone, and I am deeply obliged to and sometimes daunted by his formidable brain.

Without complaining or expectation of reward, family members painstakingly make us who we are. Reid and Ann Neilsen passed on a devotion to Civil War soldiers that is otherwise mystifying for a native Californian, while Joan Shively-Le helped provide the framework for my creative world, as all good older sisters should. Countless drops of ink have been spilled thanking life partners for their support and love in the bizarre world of academia. To Mark, I am grateful for selflessness, gentleness, and technical support far surpassing the call of duty. Along with my parents, who filled my life with books, curiosity, and love, this dedication belongs to you. The three of you share my utmost admiration.

Nature's Civil War

Introduction

Civil war changed Virginia. In 1862, the blue-green patchwork of Shenandoah Valley hills and farms and the immense, slithering rivers of the Peninsula, so picturesque from a distance, became more like sprawling latrines to the hundreds of thousands of humans who hunkered down to make war. Regiments and their horses rapidly fouled the water supplying encampments, and, in the worse cases, piled trash high between the rows of their tents, forming transitory urban slums. Armies felled trees for firewood and shelter, eliminating protection from the sun and rain, while digging entrenchments produced standing pools of water that bred mosquito larvae. The bodies of men and animals slain in battle polluted soil and air and attracted fearsome swarms of flies. In 1862, Virginia looked and felt ominous, and indeed it was.

War also changed common soldiers. The men who composed Union and Confederate armies now labored almost entirely outside, exposed to exceptionally challenging conditions with scanty protection. Too often they lacked supplies, infrastructures, and, crucially, the scientific knowledge that might have encouraged better environmental management. When illness or melancholy struck, soldiers most intensely missed civilian life; before the war, they had relied upon family members (usually women) to care for them in times of distress. Now they were expected to turn to army surgeons, whose limited understandings of disease and uneven training rendered them unreliable, their treatments suspect. Worse still, soldiers would be treated in the hospital, a space once reserved for the unloved, the itinerant, and the urban poor. The soldier became entangled in this frightening new existence before he even fired his weapon at the enemy.

Eighteen sixty-two Virginia, and indeed the Civil War as a whole, provides a window in time to when hundreds of thousands of average

Americans lifted their pens to interpret and respond to an environment they largely perceived as hostile to their survival. Indeed, both Federals and Confederates believed nature to be a significant and sometimes definitive force in shaping their physical and mental health. Connections between the body, climate, weather, seasons, terrain, flora, fauna, water, and air were so commonplace in soldier accounts that they have appeared as background rather than objects of analysis in previous histories of the common soldier. In light of the oft-quoted statistic that at least two-thirds of Civil War mortalities were from disease, these overlooked stories can help to answer a perplexing question that scholars have failed to even ask: How did any Civil War soldier remain healthy?

Stationed on the Virginia Peninsula in July, a hazardous month darkened by clouds of malaria-bearing mosquitoes, Pvt. Allen S. Davis informed his brother, rather remarkably, "My health is fine now and I enjoy myself very well and keep in the shade as much as possible. The weather is very hot but occasionally have some cooling showers. The health of the troops is improving and the army of the Potomac is in excellent spirits."[1] The Minnesotan's analysis of the interconnectivity of nature, health, morale, and behavior stemmed from his observations of the environment and lived experience in the ranks. The soldier who, like Davis, could adapt to the uniquely challenging environment of war, becoming fully "seasoned" in contemporary parlance, had a better chance of maintaining high morale and good health, proving more valuable to his unit and more likely to survive the war. Soldier adaptations, or what I term self-care, could be as simple as Davis's use of tree shelter to avoid heatstroke or range to the remarkably creative. Self-care could include eradicating pests; constructing protective shelters; intervening in camp terrain; supplementing rations, especially with fruits and vegetables; locating suitable water for drinking and bathing; attending to sanitation and dress; obtaining regular exercise; and straggling for relief. It was often a group effort; soldiers taught each other techniques or learned from officers, formed communal messes to share food, cared for one another when illness did strike, and reached out to civilians at home and at the front for advice, supplies, and comfort. What resulted was an unofficial network of care, in contrast to the military Medical Departments, which resembled the individualized and familiar health system of prewar civilian life.

Self-care was more effective at keeping soldiers fit than the official army systems, particularly in 1862, the first full calendar year of the war. In 1862 the Union and Confederate Medical Departments were still scrambling to implement adequate infrastructures. The year marked a shift when civilian aid organizations would attempt more direct interactions with soldiers, but hostility from the military often impeded intervention. The Union's official aid collective, the U.S. Sanitary Commission, of which there was no single Confederate equivalent, was most successful at integrating into the official medical system. Its middle-class reformers engaged in an immense health-education campaign among officers and surgeons and even sent inspectors into camps to analyze environmental conditions and recommend improvements to sanitation and morale. While 1862 saw major Medical Department improvements, from a Union ambulance corps to the construction of new hospitals for both sides, the soldiers of this study were only beginning to reap the benefits of reform, a slow process in democratic societies.

Further, self-care's ability to prevent illness made it superior to official army health care, a key advantage considering how poorly disease and treatment were understood. In fact, prevention was not considered the domain of nineteenth-century physicians; doctors focused instead on palliative care, which often involved chemical medications (frequently mercury-based) or heroic techniques (such as purging) that produced visible results to confirm successful cures. In short, professional remedies could be as dangerous as the diseases they were intended to alleviate. The popular conviction shared by soldiers that environment influenced illness was not so far afield of germ theory and vector-borne disease theory, major postwar intellectual advancements that would revolutionize health in the 1870s and 1880s. For example, eschewing water that tasted or smelled foul in favor of well water could prevent contact with dangerous microbes. Avoiding the perceived miasma of a swamp, or at least draining it of moisture, could prevent contact with malaria-bearing mosquitoes. Conversely, mid-century American scientists were bogged down by increasingly complex and contradictory theories of disease causation that sometimes belied observation and experience.

Additionally, self-care more directly targeted mental health than did the Medical Departments. Professional understanding of mental ailments was even dimmer than that of disease. Self-care improved morale because so much of the pervasive melancholy in the armies had to do with exhaustion from environmental effects or the suffering related to disease. Self-care mitigated exposure and reduced the likelihood that one would become ill. Self-care also improved morale because it reinforced the men's sense of democratic identity, which involved the right and responsibility to care for one's own well-being and that of one's comrades. In Jacksonian America, disease and death were companions of daily life, and yet people were expected to educate themselves about health via domestic health manuals and newspapers, manage disease environments by intervening in their landscapes, and provide care for loved ones who fell ill. These conventions of civil society carried over to the warfront and shaped soldiers' ideas about themselves. Just as before the war, self-care provided some sense of control over one's fate.

Despite the benefits of self-care, some soldiers in 1862 Virginia invested more effort in adapting to their environments than others. High literacy rates on both sides meant that most soldiers could read about self-care techniques in newspapers or gain health support through correspondence, though access to publications or mail service was not always equal.[2] Personality surely played a part, but some soldiers were also provided with better opportunities to pursue healthy habits. Some men appeared more inclined to practice self-care when granted increased mobility and independence (such as cavalrymen on horseback), while others flourished because of the good examples of their peers, officers, or surgeons. On the whole, Confederates did not benefit from what they had initially envisioned as a health advantage over Federals—their seasoning against the Southern climate. Instead, war changed environment to the extent that every soldier was vulnerable to the diseases commonly perceived as environmental in origin, such as dysentery or typhoid fever. Virginian soldiers stationed in Virginia, however, did enjoy one advantage in self-care, though perhaps not the obvious one. Rather than noticeably benefiting from a special knowledge of their environs, those who were close to home were able to more frequently straggle from the ranks to their families for an unauthorized furlough, where they could receive care, supplies, and rest, a practice known at the time as "French leave." Virginians' closeness to home may have reinforced self-care principles and networks that fell by the wayside for others.

Many soldiers who turned to the official army structures for health support learned that it was better to pursue self-care. Army surgeons and middle-class reformers quibbled over who should have access to sick and demoralized men and how they should be cared for. The U.S. Sanitary Commission collectively displayed occasional flashes of brilliance in health care, but it was also composed of individuals who frequently dismissed the concerns of enlisted men, urging them to bear up under distress as befit middle-class sentiment. In other disputes, commanders argued with regimental-level officers over whether military or medical matters should take precedence, while surgeons often felt pulled in two directions by a desire to heal the men and to assert their rank in an unfamiliar hierarchical system in a period when their expertise was being questioned. The net effect was that environmental management and common soldier health did not receive as much attention as these issues warranted. In some cases, a soldier was, in fact, better left to his own devices, perhaps avoiding a dangerous medicine. But in other cases, he might be deprived of critical aid, such as being passed over at morning sick call when in desperate need of rest or a dose of quinine, one of the few effective treatments of the period.

The men's status as volunteers (citizen soldiers) also had complex implications for the practice of self-care and for soldier health. Volunteers were historically, and justifiably, associated with poorer health than regular soldiers because of their lack of training and self-restraint.[3] Some volunteer regiments still elected their officers, who may or may not have believed that discipline paved the way to popular leadership, while some citizen soldiers simply refused to surrender the democratic freedoms they associated with civilian life. Contravening army regulations designed to protect sanitation and build morale could have disastrous consequences for volunteer regiments as the Sanitary Commission was quick to observe.[4] One inspector beholding the 87th New York's camp put it, "Camp bad. No good action on the part of captains—cooks blundering and men complaining . . . and Col. doesn't mind having his whole camp a sink [latrine]."[5] Proper latrine construction, as dictated by army regulations, was one of the more powerful indicators of a camp's salubrity. In apparent contradiction, however, loose volunteer discipline also proved vital in allowing the men the opportunity and flexibility to practice self-care. The dual nature of the volunteer spirit bred conflict between soldiers and commanders, which came to a head over the issue of straggling. Straggling not only promptly relieved environmental strain, but also enabled other types of self-care, such as foraging or locating clean water.[6] The controversy over straggling made accomplishing self-care a progressively difficult endeavor as 1862 wore on; commanders increased their vigilance over loose discipline and escalated the associated punishments.

Whether a soldier was engaged in marching or camping also had an effect on his ability to accomplish certain self-care techniques. While camping introduced the benefit of being able to intervene in one's environment to construct adequate shelter or drain the site of standing water that might attract mosquitoes, it also engendered the disadvantages of living among hundreds or thousands of other humans. Fellow soldiers contaminated water, eliminated waste too close to the tents, and spread lice where they rested. Marching avoided the pollution of stagnancy, but it also compounded exposure with exhaustion, which could lead to heat stroke, low morale, and susceptibility to disease. A soldier could march from just a few miles to more than twenty miles in a day, and his full gear—food, dining equipment, personal effects, clothing, tent, bedrolls, weapons, and ammunition—weighed about forty pounds. When he was marching in the rugged mountains of the Shenandoah Valley or the quagmires of the Peninsula, the path could be especially arduous. The longer a soldier marched, the more likely he was to cast off fundamental protective supplies, such as his winter coat, which he would regret come camp time.

Supplies were indeed vital to a soldier's ability to care for himself, and access to supplies varied considerably. Confederates were by no means the only men who suffered from the inadequacy of their provisions; Union Maj. Gen. John C. Frémont's Valley troops were probably the most undersupplied of all Civil War soldiers in 1862. The lack of fruits and vegetables in both Federal and Rebel armies led to scurvy epidemics in July. Dry food, such as the teeth-shattering Union hardtack (some of which had been left over from the Mexican-American War), lacked nutritional value, while undercooked fresh meat could be even more dangerous, causing diarrhea or dysentery, the deadliest of Civil War diseases.[7] Federals had more access to regulation uniforms, but soldiers from both sides suffered from clothing material unequal to their task. The typical flannel or wool apparel was too hot in summer and grew threadbare by winter. Those who lacked shoes, whether because of an inept quartermaster or having lost them in the mud, were vulnerable to hookworm, which enters the human body through the feet, and footsoreness. While the luckiest Federals slept in the better-ventilated Sibley tent—a tepee, eighteen feet in diameter and twelve feet high supported by a pole upon an iron tripod—their expense and cumbersome size became increasingly prohibitive in 1862. The four-man wedge tent persevered, accommodating five or six men in a space of seven square feet, while the vast majority of soldiers buttoned together half-shelters to form a dog tent or occasionally slept under the stars.[8] In winter camp, men built more durable shelters of logs and canvas with chimneys, depending on their access to material and wood. Overall, soldiers who were issued decent rations and had superior equipment fared better, but these circumstances varied so much from regiment to regiment and season to season that supplementing one's supplies became a particular goal of those practicing self-care.

Scholars have long suspected that Civil War common soldiers faced tremendous odds against remaining well, but it appears the scattered official statistics that remain have scarcely done the soldier's plight justice.[9] The evidence collected for this book is anecdotal rather than statistically significant, and yet it suggests a far sicker and demoralized soldier population than often portrayed in the literature. Using letters, diaries, and memoirs that covered the winter camp of 1861–62 to mid-August 1862, when the Union Army of the Potomac abandoned the Peninsula and its campaign for Richmond, I noted each self-reported instance of sickness, from minor headache to extended hospitalization, and each self-reported indicator of mental state, often negative phrases such as loneliness, homesickness, or "the blues," but also positive indicators. Only around fifteen percent of Confederate and Union soldiers remained physically healthy in the soldier sample, while twenty percent evinced consistently high spirits.[10] Conversely, thirty-one percent of soldiers reported debilitating and persistent sickness, which rendered them ineffective at completing their duties for long stretches of time, while another eleven percent suffered occasionally from severe illnesses. Twenty-two percent of the men consistently complained of low morale, while another twelve percent wrote of periodic plunges in their spirits. Such attitudes contributed to reduced efficacy as soldiers and increased straggling. An additional seventeen percent of soldiers, usually officers, constantly worried that their regiments were too sick and demoralized to properly function, even if they themselves remained healthy.[11] Those soldiers who did achieve fine health and spirits practiced well-varied and consistent self-care routines.

This fact should make scholars reevaluate the process of soldier seasoning as prolonged, active, and complex. In the past, historians have acknowledged what might be termed a first stage in the new recruit's progress toward becoming a seasoned soldier: surviving the initial communicable diseases of first encampment. The onslaught of measles, chickenpox, mumps, whooping cough, diphtheria, small pox, and other contagious illnesses, to which urban-born soldiers were less vulnerable given their previous exposure, affected roughly fifty percent of green soldiers.[12] Once this wave of illnesses abated, or perhaps simultaneously, the soldier also experienced the seasoning of first combat, which has also been covered by scholars.[13] This phase resulted in mental and physical toughness as the new recruit proved that he was capable of fulfilling his training. A third stage of seasoning, however, has not been previously examined by historians, and this is the process by which soldiers came to withstand illnesses and melancholy brought on by sustained exposure to army life and the environment of war. The resulting afflictions, which the soldiers perceived as environmental in causation, could be avoided or managed to some degree by self-care.

These insights raise an important problem in the literature on Civil War medicine. Until now, scholars have not undertaken a popular medical history of Civil War soldiers, because arguably it has been impossible to do so without the lens of environmental history, a new sub-discipline of Civil War studies.[14] Jim Downs's recent *Sick from Freedom*, which details the systematic failure of the United States to support the health of freed people during and after the war, is closest to this study in its ground-up approach to Civil War medicine, though it does not look at soldiers.[15] My book, then, can only be a point of departure, not a definitive answer to the considerable number of questions left on the topic of common soldier health. Because previous medical histories have been top-down analyses based on medical workers' perspectives, our understandings of soldier health have been skewed by middle- and upper-class prejudices about who got sick, under what circumstances, and how they should be treated. While the reformers of the U.S. Sanitary Commission at times openly reinforced self-care techniques, Commission workers were likewise fundamentally constrained by how their own biases framed their thinking and what the military allowed them to do.[16] By the end of the war, Sanitary Commission leadership ultimately subsumed folk healing into a larger elitist agenda that also championed class-based constitutional and racialist theories of disease.[17] While it can be difficult to locate lower-class perspectives on health, the Civil War is the perfect opportunity to do so because so many common soldiers recorded their experiences in letters and diaries. Indeed, social history has far from run its course in bringing to light new insights into Civil War medicine.

By drawing soldiers into the conversation regarding their own health, this book attempts to reinvigorate the stalled field of common soldier studies, a tremendously popular branch of military history of the Civil War. Scholars of the common soldier have investigated soldier religion, ideology, politics, and experiences in camp, on the march, and in combat, but without asking why the men meticulously assessed their surroundings.[18] The neglect is understandable given that soldier expositions on nature often make up the most quotidian and tedious portions of wartime accounts. It is quite common for soldier letters or diaries to read as mere catalogues of weather, illness, and rations drawn. But Frances Clarke's recent *War Stories* has encouraged us to reconsider our disregard of the trivialities of soldier life. For instance, Clarke reveals that letter writing—in this study a crucial component of self-care—was a vital window into mid-century attempts to cope with suffering.[19] Several works on soldier morale have also pointed to environmental hardships as a cause of diminished soldier performance, though most have focused on the battlefield.[20] And some recent works have included soldiers in their insightful analyses of popular views on death.[21] Soldiers were, indeed, very concerned with how they would meet their demise, fearing death by disease as far less honorable than death on the battlefield. Thus, managing the environment that shaped disease became a primary preoccupation of soldiers outside of combat and deserves more investigation.

Environmental history has provided the lens for this study, and it was Conevery Bolton Valencius's astute *The Health of the Country* that first made apparent the connection between environment and health in mid-century America. Valencius revealed that antebellum Americans believed air, water, and places had crucial impacts on their bodies; and yet, by cultivation and management, one could potentially avoid becoming ill in the insalubrious regions of the South and West. Though she did not discuss mental health or the Civil War, Valencius did put the wheels in motion for this study.[22] Until recently, environmental historians have typically skipped over the Civil War as a formative moment in the development of American environmental thought.[23] This book should lend more fuel to the argument that the Civil War forced a crisis of interaction between humans and nature, testing antebellum hypotheses and driving changes in how Americans addressed their surroundings.[24]

As a first attempt to correct for considerable gaps in the literature, this work is a case study. Avid readers of soldier accounts will recognize the habits and sentiments outlined here as present throughout the time and space of the Civil War, while also noting the limitations of the year and the places I chose. The 1862 Peninsula and Shenandoah Valley campaigns did provide an appealing opportunity for research controls. They took place in approximately the same time period and roughly 200 miles apart. Maj. Gen. Thomas "Stonewall" Jackson's Valley army even joined the Peninsula campaign after achieving victory in the Shenandoah, providing single-soldier perspectives on both locales. The Valley and the Peninsula were both close to the two nations' capitals, allowing for similar political interference and higher scrutiny by the public and War Departments. The campaigns were strategically linked, and therefore what happened in one campaign influenced the other. The eastern theater was also within the most developed logistical networks, meaning soldiers had as fair a chance of being well supplied in these campaigns as they did anywhere in 1862. But just as important, I selected the two campaigns for their contrasting environments: the Peninsula was contemporarily considered a virulent disease environment for its festering swamps, while the Shenandoah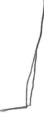

Valley was known as a health Eden. This contrast would reveal if soldiers responded to different disease environments with different attitudes and sets of behaviors.

Despite the fact that I chose the Peninsula and Valley for their conflicting environmental reputations, both locales proved hostile to soldier health and morale, and soldiers in both locations developed identical self-care regimens. Although disease was less common in the Shenandoah Valley than in the Peninsula before the war, the circumstances of constant exposure, inadequate clothing and shelter, poor rations, overcrowded campsites, deficient sanitation, and a general lack of people and institutions who had guarded health in peacetime had somewhat of a leveling effect on landscapes.[25] The Peninsula produced only slightly sicker soldiers, and even these results are skewed by the fact that the campaign was of longer duration and involved larger armies than the Shenandoah Valley campaign.[26] Further, the Valley was more dangerous to health than the Peninsula in the spring because of mercurial weather, while the mosquito-riddled Peninsula proved more threatening in the summer.[27] Though many soldiers continued to rhetorically admire the Valley, they lamented their suffering there just the same as on the Peninsula and developed the same adaptations. The fact that soldiers stationed in these strikingly different landscapes adopted a universal set of habits when faced with environmental stress suggests that Virginia is at least a suitable starting point for understanding self-care in the war at large.

The year 1862 is also ideal for investigating the seasoning process of common soldiers. The bulk of the armies in this study had moved on from the early seasoning phase, involving communicable diseases, to focus upon the illnesses they perceived as largely or partially environmental in origin: in particular, typhoid and malarial fevers, diarrhea and dysentery, rheumatism, scurvy, sunstroke, and mental ailments, such as homesickness, melancholy, and nostalgia.[28] Further, choosing an early point in the war ensures that soldiers would still describe the novelty of their situation but were also well on their way to becoming veterans. Finally, the year 1862 allows a perspective on popular conceptions of environment and health before commanders could institutionalize paternalistic responses to what they perceived as the problem and its solution. By the end of the year, military leaders chose to concentrate upon eradicating straggling, a major component of self-care. Because the material conditions of the troops were improving, it appeared to command that the major cause of straggling had been corrected; now they needed only to enforce discipline to curb the practice.[29]

That I chose to weave together Confederate and Union soldiers' stories is in itself a contentious approach to common soldier history, as much of the newer literature presents Southerners and Northerners as essentially distinct.[30] Yet the environment of war was a universalizing factor for soldiers. Both Union and Confederate troops perceived and adapted to Virginia in the same ways, recognizing the same inherent natural threats and the same solutions to their problems. I locate this commonality in the men's antebellum ideas about how human bodies interacted with nature as well as the shared experience of soldering. Further, Virginia was just as alien to a New Yorker as to a Texan. Indeed, the more apt comparison than Northerners to Southerners is between Virginians (who compose twenty-five percent of the soldiers sampled) and non-Virginians.

At the center of this book is a sample of common soldier letters, diaries, and memoirs from the winter of 1861–62 to mid-August 1862 when the Peninsula campaign came to a close.[31] Seventy-five percent were enlisted men, because they constituted the majority of war experience and faced more extreme environmental exposure than did the higher ranks. Around eighty-seven percent were in the infantry compared with a small sample of the other army branches, including five percent cavalry and seven percent artillery. Further, surgeons are included in the sample (seven percent overall), because they, too, had to undergo seasoning and were, at times, very ill.[32] Some surgeons also practiced self-care techniques. Seventy-six percent of the evidential base is composed of soldiers' diaries and letters, while the remaining twenty-four percent are memoirs. Even though many of the memoirists in this sample based their accounts on their diaries or letters, it is, as usual, important to bear in mind the differences between eyewitness accounts and retrospectives.[33] Memoirists did not always reflect their wartime experiences and attitudes accurately. Nineteenth-century Americans feared being labeled as cowardly or self-pitying, particularly by their families, who would be sure to read their memoirs.[34] Retrospective accounts are therefore mainly used to determine self-care techniques the soldiers recalled using, the experiences and people they deemed important to survival, and their persistent interest in environmental health, as some soldiers wished to recast their wartime experiences in terms of late-century scientific discoveries. Further, memoirs help to locate accounts of straggling, which soldiers often left out of eyewitness records for fear of being caught and punished.

This story belongs to the soldiers of 1862. Those people who played critical roles in shaping soldier health—such as generals, medical directors, and civilians—appear only as supporting characters. The military and medical command perspective on environmental management and health is established using the *Official Records* and documents from the War Departments, as well as personal accounts from generals, government officials, and medical directors. I use official medical data from *The Medical and Surgical History of the War of the Rebellion*, Confederate regimental records, Joseph Janvier Woodward's *Outlines of the Chief Camp Diseases of the United States Armies*, medical journals, newspapers, and the U.S. Sanitary Commission, but bearing in mind their serious limitations. Army regulations are determined by training manuals, general orders, and the *Official Records*. The civilian perspective and contributions to self-care are constructed from newspapers, letters, and diaries, and the personal papers and published works of the U.S. Sanitary Commission. Antebellum and wartime medical professional debates appeared in medical journals, newspapers, and published texts.

Applying the subfield of environmental history to the Civil War is a relatively new endeavor and one that requires a brief explication of terms. Nature is a word that has been so debated by environmental historians that it is only useful when defined in its particular contexts. In this text, nature is a synonym for environment: non-human, non-manmade ecological, meteorological, and topographical phenomena, including the related set of weather, seasons, and climate, as well as air, water, terrain, insects, animals, and plant life. The only diseases and mental afflictions investigated are those that soldiers deemed fully or partially environmental in origin, and I include only those that occurred in 1862 Virginia. I do, however, engage with both environmental and non-environmental solutions to these perceived environmental problems. For example, a soldier could seek a natural preventative, such as foraging for berries as a barrier against scurvy, or he could seek a remedy for depressed spirits after days of lying out in the rain by writing a letter home to connect with a loved one.

Most important to this study are soldier perceptions of environment and the self-care they devised as a response, but I also occasionally weigh the benefits of their actions against modern scientific understandings of disease. I do so not to engage in presentism, but rather to demonstrate the real efficacy of self-care in preserving health, thereby explaining why those who practiced self-care tended to remain healthy and in better spirits. Mental health is particularly hard to investigate, but soldiers did suggest fairly direct causal links between environmental threats and diminished spirits.[35] I took note of each time a solider linked environment to feeling "homesick," "depressed," "lonesome," or having "the blues." Civil War surgeons also employed the term "nostalgia" to describe a potentially fatal brand of homesickness accompanied by fever, gastrointestinal distress, headache, weeping, and even hallucinations. These symptoms could have been hallmarks of malaria or other physical ailments, symptoms of severe distress, or perhaps both. When taken on the larger scale and put into military parlance, we might understand these mental states to be diminished morale, which limited army operations. This study, then, serves as another reminder that we as military historians must continue to look beyond the battlefield to understand fluctuations in morale.[36]

As a final point of reference, it is important to consider breaking the habit of divorcing mental from physical health. Nineteenth-century Americans may have entertained a simpler, more direct view of nature's ability to upend the body than germ theory, but they also possessed a more complex understanding of the interconnectedness of body, mind, and environment. This perception appears justified by the evidence, as soldiers who suffered frequently from sickness often, in turn, became melancholic and dejected.[37] Losing so many comrades to environmental illness also made men despondent, lonely, and fearful for their futures. Further, contemporaries believed that attitude affected physical well-being: a negative attitude could weaken a person or prevent healing, while a positive spirit could result in recovery. Again, this view was not insupportable by observation. Optimistic soldiers tended to practice self-care while the resigned often did not.

This book, then, at its core is an ethnographic history of soldier health. For all the novelty war brought, soldiers were products of their upbringings and the Jacksonian era; therefore, chapter 1 briefly lays out prewar popular understandings of mental and physical health in contrast and sometimes in unison with the views of the emerging professionals and middle-class reformers who would construct the official wartime systems of health care. Laypeople put the most stock in what they could observe and intuit, favoring environmental explanations of illness, while doctors and reformers competed for popular confidence in additional theories. Future common soldiers had also developed personal networks of health care that they were reluctant to abandon once in uniform and would attempt to recreate in 1862.

Chapter 2 plunges into soldier experience in 1862, as the bulk of men had already been seasoned by crowd diseases, freeing them to focus primarily on the ailments they considered environmental in origin. Surprisingly, the experience of being at war with nature appeared to be universal for Confederate and Union soldiers, regardless of where they were from, because war changed the land from its antebellum state and soldiers were more vulnerable to exposure. Many of the men's preconceptions about seasoning were tested, while other ideas were confirmed. The soldiers were not completely unarmed in their fight for survival in the elements, as chapter 3 explores; they were part of an official network of health care developed by their respective Medical Departments. The Union and Confederate war machines busily set about constructing sprawling and impressive health systems that would reduce the number of disease mortalities at war's end from the staggering eighty percent of the Mexican-American War to just sixty-six percent. And yet, 1862 was a year of trial, failure, and reinvention in terms of infrastructure, and soldiers were unaccustomed to professional care. Because of this reality, the troops were highly suspicious and critical of a system that seemed indifferent to their comfort and inadequate to the task of keeping them alive. In response to both their heightened susceptibility to wartime disease environments and their dissatisfaction with the Medical Departments, chapter 4 explains that soldiers constructed their own networks of environmental knowledge and health care outside of the military establishment. Soldiers devised self-care routines based on prewar and wartime experience, the guidance and care of fellow soldiers, and the advice of civilians in and around the camps—often women and African Americans—and those who were more distant but communicated through newspapers and correspondence. Self-care often demonstrably improved physical health and morale.

The military is a system that relies upon regimentation and hierarchy, and so the soldiers' unofficial health care networks could not survive for long without falling under the scrutiny of their superiors. Therefore, chapter 5 examines the controversy that erupted over the erosion of discipline that self-care engendered, epitomized by the practice of straggling. As command increasingly punished straggling, they also allowed disciplinary concerns to surpass their disquiet over ballooning sickness and faltering morale. The campaigns of this study thus ended at a critical crossroads: when the Army of the Potomac abandoned the Peninsula, in part because of excessive sickness in the ranks, and Robert E. Lee did very much the same.[38] Straggling predictably climaxed that fall, but by winter commanders finally asserted their disciplinary agendas to greater success. The shape of soldier self-care would perhaps have to change, with 1863 also promising more robust official medical infrastructures. Weathering that first year and a half of war, however, remained very much to the credit of common soldiers.

Finally, a few words on what this book does not do. This is not a story about surgery, a much-storied aspect of Civil War medicine. In fact, the content of these pages should prompt us to consider why we continue to preserve the contemporary bias that favored attention to surgery over the more frequent killer, disease. Likewise, this is not a story about combat, but rather a story about what happened during the majority of soldier life in between the spaces of battles. The book is both limited and facilitated by its case study and calls for a follow-up inquiry in the later stages of the war to assess if soldiers made progress on self-care or if they were permanently hampered by the increased regulation of their daily lives. It is also a social history and may even emphasize soldiers' individual attempts to survive to a fault, given that so much of military success has to do with orderliness and sacrifice.

Despite the persistent romanticizing of our nation's Civil War by American culture, there can be no doubt: soldiering was a miserable business. And yet common soldiers, in spite of many of their low-class origins and the tremendous limitations of army life, constructed startlingly effective networks of environmental knowledge and health care. In a system predicated upon responsibility being yielded up the chain of command, it was still the individual who cared most for his own survival. Sgt. Shepard Pryor of Georgia wrote his sweetheart with poignant honesty: "That is what I dread most in the service is getting sick in camp. I fear if I was to get bad sick in camp it would kill me."[39] Each man thus lived with the hope that if he died he would go quickly on the battlefield, not alone after the prolonged agony of a sickness he only dimly understood but acutely suffered,

I

Health and the American Populace before 1862

In their wartime journals and correspondence, soldiers fixated upon cataloging their natural environments. Pvt. William Randolph Smith of the 17th Virginia, for example, wrote in March 1862, "There is the finest pine timber on the road I ever saw. . . . The farms are also fine and fertile. . . . From Robison River to the Rapidan is the finest country I ever saw. The land is easily cultivated and is splendid." He also recorded the weather with painstaking precision: "We had some fine weather on the march, but some very bad. Tuesday, Wednesday, and Thursday, the 11th, and 12th, and 13th were very fine. Then it was rainy and quite disagreeable camping out without any protection, from the rain until the 16th when we had some fine days until the 19th when the Equinoctial rains commenced and continued without remissions until the 2nd when it cleared away, and the weather is now clear and cool." On March 28, he lowered his keen gaze earthward. "The ground is full of stumps but lays well, and have an abundance of water, which is so essential to the soldiers health."[1] Such fastidious (even tedious) detail is not simply an idle soldier's Civil War Era small talk—it presents continuity with his farming roots. Smith identified land that could be easily cultivated, catalogued the exact dates of precipitation, and connected environment to human health. Like Smith, the majority of soldiers were farmers with extensive experience observing nature, because environmental circumstances shaped their livelihoods and, they believed, their health.[2] They connected the visible changes in nature, which governed planting and harvesting, to the invisible worlds of their bodies and minds. Even the smaller population of Americans who grew up in cities was accustomed to the idea that environment—the

crowds and filth by which urbanites were surrounded—contributed 、
diseases.

Explaining disease origins based on observation and experience made
more sense to average Americans than parsing out new, often conflicting scientific theories. While most Americans were literate and could
read about the scientific debates raging among orthodox physicians and
middle-class reformers, they exhibited a clear preference for self-reliance
typical of the Jacksonian era.[3] After all, the 1840s push toward medical professionalization, epitomized by the establishment of the American Medical Association in 1847, did not mean doctors proved better at
rescuing Americans from the clutches of death. Historian Mark Schantz
estimates that the quarter century preceding the war actually brought a
dip in life expectancy; average Americans only lived to their mid-forties.[4]
Doctors provided diagnoses and medications but left comfort and care
to one's family members. Furthermore, access to professional physicians
was limited, particularly in rural and developing areas, such as the South
and the West. For these reasons, antebellum laypeople interacted infrequently with medical experts and developed their own means of transmitting medical knowledge, but the Civil War would usher in a cultural shift
that pushed common soldiers into contact with physicians, reformers,
and hospitals.[5] Because soldiers in 1862 attempted to retain and recreate
prewar health ideas and care networks in the midst of great challenges to
civilian norms, it is important to understand the antebellum health experience before turning to the war.

DISEASE ENVIRONMENTS OF
THE EARLY NINETEENTH CENTURY

While there was a dizzying array of hypotheses about what caused mental
and physical sickness, historian Conevery Bolton Valencius has identified
common ground among Jacksonian Americans when it came to conceiv-
ing of disease environments. Prevailing ideas followed several trends.
First, different geographic regions produced distinctive diseases, which
also varied based on the seasons and weather. The surest way to avoid an
environmental illness was to physically relocate, if one were able. Second, bodies underwent a process of seasoning, or bodily adjusting to a
new climate when one moved, which is something most soldiers would
experience in wartime. Because migration characterized the antebellum
period as well, Valencius explains that Americans frequently discussed
the salubrity of places, considering the seasoning process "debilitating

ng."[6] Sometimes entering a new area could so profoundly
as to trigger mental infirmity— "hysteria, hypochondria
is one medical journal cautioned.[7] Accordingly, itinerant
vell schooled in examining the weather, water, air, and
markers of a place. Third, specific terrain features within a cer-
in area influenced disease but could potentially be altered to mitigate
their impacts. Americans used agricultural and irrigation techniques to
assert control over potentially hostile environments. Farmers were instructed to drain marshes and wetlands and to allow trees to stand by
lakes, rivers, and ponds as barriers against miasmatic air.[8] Indeed, tam-
ing the wilderness to disarm its threats had been a theme of American
settlement for hundreds of years.[9]

The first concept—that certain regions produced certain diseases—
requires a bit more explanation, as it would prove vastly influential upon
Civil War soldier thinking. Not only were all people considered products
of their particular environment—and thus seasoned to a specific geography and population density—but most soldiers would ultimately be stationed in the South, and in this study, in Virginia. Chilly, mountainous
regions (such as those common to the North) were considered detrimental
to the respiratory system, harming sufferers of tuberculosis or pneumonia.
Alternatively, lowland, hot, and humid areas with truncated winters and
swamps (such as those common to the South) earned reputations even
by residents as particularly conducive to "fevers"—a generic category that
encompassed a number of diseases that produced the symptom, such as
malaria and typhoid—and bowel disorders. Modern historians have likewise noted the "epidemiological distinctiveness" of regions where diseases
of African origin, such as multiple malarial parasites, yellow fever, and
hookworm, flourished.[10] Contemporarily, Hippocrates's *On Airs, Waters
and Places* had long postulated that the air of wet, poorly drained terrain
conducted disease, and the related miasma theory suggested that swamps
emitted harmful vapors that could be identified by their putrid smells.[11]
When ill, Southerners of means often traveled in search of cooler climes to
foster recovery.[12] Avoiding dank areas could be surprisingly effective given
that this reduced exposure to malaria-carrying mosquitoes. Thus, positive
health results appeared to confirm the miasma theory and had kept it alive
for centuries. The miasma theory certainly appeared substantiated when
soldiers descended upon Virginia in 1862, resulting in massive outbreaks
of malaria, typhoid fever, dysentery, and diarrhea. Indeed, Confederates
hoped that their acclimated bodies would prove stronger than those of
unseasoned Federals, but they were wrong.[13]

In prewar Virginia, life-threatening malaria tied the border area in with the Deep South rather than the Northern states. There are actually four types of plasmodia that cause malaria—vivax, falciparum, malarie, and ovale—and the most common, vivax, could thrive to some degree in both cool and warmer climes. Its symptoms included the telltale fevers and potential anemia common to all types of malaria. While it lay dormant in the liver and could recur indefinitely, its ultimate consequences tended to be relatively minor. Mortalities usually occurred only among the immune-compromised or malnourished. In contrast, the deadliest form of malaria, produced by the falciparum plasmodia, lived exclusively in climates south of Pennsylvania. It was carried to America in the bodies of Africans, perhaps a quarter of whom had a sickle-cell trait that granted them diminished susceptibility and lower mortality rates, leading to a widespread belief that enslaved people could better endure the Southern climate.[14] Besides producing fevers and anemia in its host, the Falciparum plasmodium could trigger epilepsy, blindness, cognitive impairment, behavioral disturbances, coma, and even death in twenty-five to fifty percent of victims if left untreated. Once cured, however, victims completely recovered and enjoyed future immunity, again appearing to confirm the idea of seasoning.[15] Because malaria was so common in Virginia, the state gained a reputation as a potentially fearsome disease environment, much like its Southern neighbors. Once war enveloped the area, Virginia's variable weather and large expanses of swamp would further conduct the diseases common to armies, such as typhoid fever, transmitted through feces-contaminated water.

There was also an antebellum conception of the city as a sicklier environment than the country. One 1840 newspaper article, "Importance of Pure Air," explained that parents should take special care to help their children avoid crowds. "At this tender and susceptible period of life, the rapid influence of the atmosphere in which we live, in deteriorating or improving the health, is very remarkable, a change of a few weeks from the country to a large town being sufficient to change the ruddy, healthy child into a pale, sickly-looking creature." Indeed, "Children should never be reared in large towns when this can be avoided; and, when unavoidable, they should be sent during a part, at least, of every summer into the country."[16] Americans who had grown up in cities had very often been seasoned by childhood diseases, such as scarlatina or diphtheria, and epidemics, such as cholera, consumption, and yellow fever. Their resulting vast experience with death and its accompanying piles of fly-speckled bodies lining the streets prompted historian Mark Schantz's comment that "such scenes of mass death, burial trenches, and refugees call to mind parallels with Civil War battlefields."[17] The nuances of the urban-specific disease environment actually produced considerable confusion once the Civil War came. Many soldiers predicted that country boys would prove heartier than city boys, when in fact rural Americans were exposed for the first time to crowd diseases, making them more likely to become ill than those who had survived epidemics as children.

All soldiers and caretakers involved in the Peninsula and Shenandoah Valley campaigns would have to confront their preconceptions about disease regions contained in Virginia. Before the war, Virginia was largely rural, but during the war it would be experienced as an urban environment. Before the war, the Peninsula and Shenandoah Valley environments were also considered distinct—the Peninsula a hazardous swampland and the Shenandoah Valley a fertile agricultural landscape. During the war they would become comparably insalubrious.

Many prewar medical journal articles cautioned Americans against even entering Southern swamps, such as those located on the Peninsula. For instance, in June of 1843, several authors from the *Western Journal of Medicine* denounced Alabamian and Mississippian wetlands. In their month-long travels, they had "snuffed up the exhalations of swamps . . . in sufficient numbers to supply malaria for a continent, and raise a smile of complacent satisfaction on the lip of every advocate of the malarious origin of congestive fever."[18] Dr. Charles Lucas of the *American Journal of the Medical Sciences* postulated in the Hippocratic vein that standing water generated miasma. "The sluggish and frequently stagnant waters of these lagoons, exposed to the intense and continued action of a scorching sun, are soon covered with a green scum, are the nidus of myriads of insects, and the surrounding atmosphere speedily becomes offensively tainted." Lucas went on, in typical fashion for the period, to encode the landscape of health in racial terms. "Negroes . . . reside during the intense heat of summer in the most sickly situations, with the utmost perfect impunity, while the whites are obliged to retire in order to avoid the deleterious influence of the miasms."[19] During the Civil War, "whites" would not have the option to retreat from the swamps in the summer and fall, forcing them to confront their fears about miasma.

As suggested by Lucas, Americans perceived the environmental dangers of the swamps as being cyclical in nature, a concept seemingly reinforced by the periodic suffering of vivax victims. One doctor who investigated Virginia in 1823 noted that while "tertians" (a term that usually referred to vivax malaria) were frequent in April through October where wet ground was abundant, the winter wind's "effect was so remarkable in sweeping off these fevers, that it was a common observation when the first north west wind came, to say, the Doctor is come now, and we shall soon get well."[20] The problem in wartime was that most active campaigning would take place precisely during what proved the sickliest months of the year: April to November.

The Shenandoah Valley, which was free from swamps and more mountainous in terrain, was alternatively viewed as a healthful region before the war. Indeed, modern studies suggest there was less diarrhea, only vivax malaria, and no hookworm, if slightly more respiratory ailments.[21] In one antebellum article promoting the Valley's salubrity, Dr. James Thomson encouraged more exploration of the Valley's geography, citing its bounty of medicinal plants, mineral springs, and specifically the "tonic and laxative" waters near Harpers Ferry. As a cure for "bilious cases," he noted that "these waters have proved highly beneficial—correcting debility by imparting a vigorous tone to the stomach, whose sympathetic influence is speedily felt throughout the system." Indeed, many healers recommended soaking in the waters of the Valley or breathing in its mountain air. Despite the preference for the Valley's climate, even it proved occasionally unhealthy in a time when little about disease causation was well understood. Valley residents had recently experienced two "calamitous seasons" of intermittent and remittent fever, which Thomson attributed to "certain changes which take place in the atmosphere, not cognisable to the sense, produced by heat and moisture evolving noxious exhalations, from the decomposition of vegetable matter principally—that these exhalations partake of the nature of the soil, temperature, and seasons in which they are generated."[22] The fact that fevers (and most likely malaria) were not always neatly confined to the lowlands produced some contemporary puzzlement, leading to continued investigation by so-called medical topographers, or physicians who investigated disease landscapes by collecting data through observation and interviews with locals.[23] Thomson, for instance, located miasma not only in the common explanations of swamps and rotting vegetable matter but also in atmospheric shifts (another environmental explanation), which seemed to comport with the variable weather common to the Valley.

Americans of all social classes often subscribed to the concepts of disease environments and seasoning, but the lower classes particularly favored environmental explanations because they seemed to be confirmed by lived experience. While average Americans did not tend to expound upon their medical opinions in the antebellum period, enlisted soldiers would frequently do so during the Civil War, providing a window into popular medical thought that had not previously existed.

AVERAGE AMERICANS AND SELF-CARE

Average Americans developed a discernible set of health-related behaviors and beliefs common to their class that would shape their actions in wartime. For instance, most Americans had rare contact with doctors, especially those from rural areas, while it was a prerogative of the rich to travel for medical advice. Home was the primary venue of recovery in times of illness, where family members, most often mothers, sisters, and wives, provided care rather than cure.[24] Historian Jane Schultz encapsulates it best: "Every woman was a nurse."[25] Care was an intimate affair administered in one's own bed. A sick person engrossed the entire family, who could not escape the sights, smells, and sounds of infirmity.[26] Because disease was not well understood, death was a far more common outcome from even moderate illnesses, provoking tremendous anxiety and religious fervor. The prevalence of home care meant that few Americans had experience with hospitals. Hospitals, located almost exclusively in cities, were for the destitute, those who lacked family, or those who were, perhaps, outsiders traveling in a foreign city.[27]

While achieving good health was in many ways a collective undertaking, there was also a widespread ethos of taking responsibility for one's own body. Though self-care had always been a part of human experience, Jacksonian Americans particularly embraced the spirit of self-reliance as befit the democratic age.[28] In a predominantly literate culture, they had wide access to do-it-yourself medical books, newspapers, and medical journals. Many reformers, some even trained physicians, actively sought to engage the common person in his or her own health care, giving rise to the phenomenon of the domestic medicine manual, which quickly became a staple in American households. Women often proved the dispensers of such knowledge, sometimes authoring or compiling their own recipe books of remedies.[29]

One of the earliest household manuals was William Buchan's *Domestic Medicine*, a product of the Scottish enlightenment. The book could be found in most American homes, though its popularity waned slightly in the 1820s, to be replaced by a homegrown American version.[30] It covered a vast array of ailments and suggested responsive curative "regimens" and simple "medical preparations," using accessible language. Buchan meant to correct the fact that "the generality of people lay too much stress upon

Medicine, and trust too little their own endeavors." Not only did he celebrate the layperson's experiential knowledge, but he granted them access to alleged medical secrets by proposing that "the cure of diseases does not depend so much upon scientific principles. By attending and observing the various occurrences in diseases, a great degree of accuracy may be acquired in distinguishing their symptoms, and in the application of medicines."[31] Each person could act as his or her physician, as long as the person was observant, relieving the need in most cases for ever calling upon a doctor.

The American version of the domestic manual was *Gunn's Domestic Medicine*, alternatively (and appropriately) titled *Poor Man's Friend, in the Hours of Affliction, Pain, and Sickness*. First published in 1830, it gained extensive popularity and was reprinted more than 200 times up into the twentieth century.[32] While originally meant to inform rural people in Tennessee how to care for themselves in isolation, it also served as a guide for self-taught country doctors. The manual's extensive subtitle from the 1860 edition spelled out the philosophy behind domestic manuals: "This book points out, in plain language, free from doctor's terms, the diseases of men, women, and children, and the latest and most approved means used in their cure, and is intended expressly for the benefit of families." It reduced the practice of medicine to "common sense." For "why should we conceal from mankind that which relieves the distresses of our fellow-beings?" the subtitle pondered. The maladies included in the book covered everything from "bowel complaint" to cancer to grief to hysteria—displaying attention to both physical and mental conditions—and remedies from beer to ginseng to do-it-yourself bloodletting. Among its many cures, it more often emphasized natural solutions and contained "descriptions of the medicinal roots and herbs of the United States, and how they are to be used in the cure of diseases."[33] Soldiers did not bring this hefty manual to the front nor did they directly reference it, but its knowledge and spirit were diffuse.

More examples of the prewar self-care literature included the monthly periodical the *Water Cure Journal* (*WCJ*) and other similar publications. The journal was geared, at least in part, toward the public. Advertisements for the journal ran in everything from the *New York Evening Post* to African American newspapers, such as the *National ERA*. The *WCJ* was touted as "unquestionably, the most popular health journal in the world." Its articles by the "ablest medical writers" dealt with "all subjects relating to the Laws of Life, Health, and Happiness." It advertised as "published monthly, illustrated with Engravings, exhibiting the structure, anatomy, and physiology of the human body, with familiar instructions to learners.

It is . . . designed to be a complete Family Guide in all diseases." Not only was the *WCJ* affordable for the masses at one dollar per year, but, like much of the domestic care literature, it emphasized the family as the unit where treatment should rightly take place.[34] It provided the tools necessary for learning about and understanding the human body.

Newspapers, also consumed by the masses, likewise ran articles on disease prevention and cure. To pick up the story of the article mentioned earlier that directed parents to raise their children in the countryside rather than the city, the author—Dr. James Clarke—explicitly saw himself as the mediator of life-saving knowledge between professionals and lay people. "We have reason to believe that the advantages of country air to the young and delicate are not yet sufficiently appreciated by the profession; and we are, therefore, anxious to call their attention to it, that they may use their influence with the public . . . [to] contribut[e] greatly to the health of the rising generation."[35] Because Clarke believed medical professionals to be slow to appreciate his theory of disease causation, he decided it best to bypass his colleagues in favor of appealing directly to the people. Clarke was one of a number of professionals who published in the popular media in an attempt to manage public health.

All in all, average Americans were savvy and proactive about collecting information on their bodies. They took individual and collective responsibility for their own health and that of their loved ones, understanding that the consequences of sickness were all too often death. Home care and do-it-yourself remedies were, in many cases, as effective—or perhaps better put, as ineffective—as professional medicine, considering the state of scientific knowledge. But the comfort of care provided by loved ones could not be matched by that of doctors or hospitals.

PHYSICIANS AND ORTHODOX MEDICINE

Before the war, laypeople had relatively few interactions with traditional (or orthodox) doctors, except when it came to surgery or more complex cases of illness that required professional diagnosis. Yet because professional physicians would soon have profound impacts upon survival during the Civil War, as they constituted the majority of surgeons, it is important to realize that traditional medical authority was in a period of decline. This resulted in many orthodox doctors re-entrenching in therapeutic philosophies that overvalued dramatic medical interventions, made assumptions about the health of the lower classes, and excluded preventative techniques.

In the antebellum period, the traditional physician's identity derived from experience rather than a special claim to scientific expertise. Medical colleges and universities were sparse and lacked standardization, thus apprenticeship remained an accepted means of acquiring training. In medical historian John Harley Warner's assessment, a physician's reputation was built upon his practical knowhow, personal character, and interaction with patients. In short, his personal reputation was his professional identity.[36] This is an important distinction to make from modern physicians, who might be measured by the success of their treatments. As scholar Stephen Halliday has stressed, virtually no universal understanding of disease, save smallpox, existed in the period.[37] One might also add scurvy to the list of hazily understood and treatable illnesses, as most professionals recognized that adding vegetables and fruits to the diet could help to prevent and cure the disease, though medical literature from the Civil War demonstrates lingering confusion on the topic.[38] Further, cinchona bark and its synthetic cousin quinine were widely regarded as effective treatments for malaria when properly administered; however, they were hardly the only substances proscribed for fevers.[39]

The challenge to traditional medicine, beginning in earnest in the 1820s, came from within the field by sectarianism and without by democratic society.[40] Over time, a new class of young, aspiring physicians began emphasizing medical school education, instruction abroad in France, and scientific experimentation in contrast to the old, "rational" school.[41] Further, practitioners of new therapeutic techniques, particularly homeopaths, successfully pushed for the state-level repeal of medical licensing laws.[42] Without a distinct educational path or certifying system, orthodox practitioners had little to distinguish their expertise from those they considered quacks. Thus, traditional doctors sought to carve out their distinct sphere by emphasizing the highly visible nature of their treatments, especially heroic interventions.[43]

Heroic medicine involved the conception of four main bodily fluids, called "humors": blood, phlegm, yellow bile (or choler), and black bile. The humors were sometimes linked to the seasons of the year (spring, summer, autumn, and winter) and to the seasons of life (childhood, youth, adulthood, and old age). Treatment revolved around Galen's expression of humors as fluids in need of balance, which could be achieved by visibly expelling blood, pus, vomit, diarrhea, and sweat.[44] To these ends, popular medications included antiphlogistics, which instigated sweating to break fevers; purgatives or cathartics, which induced diarrhea with low-level mercury; emetics, which precipitated vomiting; opium or morphine,

which increased the appetite and reduced pain; skin irritants or canthari-
des, which evacuated pus; and healing tonics and quinine.[45] While earlier Hippocratic theory had also emphasized the patient's ability to self-
repair without interference, antebellum doctors swept aside this wisdom
in their pursuit of professionalization. Most doctors regarded an external
symptom as the disease itself.[46] It thus appeared that medical treatment
was effective only when it produced noticeable changes in the symptom,
even if that change was for the worse. Many of the heroic treatments were
not well received among the populace, who considered them invasive and
unpleasant. While the practice of bleeding declined in response, heroic
stimulation actually peaked during the Civil War years, particularly when
it came to the use of mercury-based medications.[47] Further, none of the
heroic treatments were preventative, except in the case of the smallpox
vaccine.[48]

Humoral theory had implications for connecting physical and mental
health, and yet diagnosis and treatment often followed a highly scripted,
narrow path. The four humors were often linked to temperaments—the sanguine, choleric/bilious, melancholic/nervous, and phlegmatic/lymphatic—
as a component of constitutional pathology. Under this line of thinking,
certain constitutions, which could be identified by the physical appearance
of a person, were deemed heartier, such as the sanguine and the choleric,
while the melancholic and phlegmatic were more prone to disease. Each
type, however, was predisposed to certain ailments. For instance, a sanguine
person was believed to expend most of the blood in his or her youth, making
the person more vigorous and attractive early on but more likely to die pre-
maturely. The sanguine were more susceptible to moral and dietetic lapses
and the associated venereal diseases, madness, and diabetes. Those of a
bilious makeup tended toward indigestion, liver problems, and the mental
suite of depression, hypochondria, and melancholy. The nervous type was
most susceptible to hysteria, addiction, and epilepsy. The lymphatic possessed high pain thresholds but would likely die of disease—perhaps gout,
diarrhea, or childhood diseases, such as scarlatina. Each temperament had
preferred treatments, such as depressants for the sanguine, mercury for the
bilious, opiates for the melancholy, and cathartics for the lymphatic.[49]

Constitutional theory quickly progressed beyond benign categorization
to facilitate class-based, racial, and ethnic stereotypes that would remain
in place during the Civil War. Organizing humans according to bodily
features, mental health, and intellect became increasingly popular in the
wake of the publication of Charles Darwin's theory of evolution in 1859.
Darwin himself contacted the U.S. military during the Civil War in the

hopes of acquiring statistics that might link soldiers' physical attributes to tropical diseases. Along these same lines, insurance companies underwrote a considerable amount of the U.S. Sanitary Commission's expenses during the war, convinced that the statistics collected on Union soldiers would yield better information about the premiums that could be charged based on buyers' appearances.[50] Medical lessons of the Civil War would by no means stamp out this strain of thinking; indeed, many of the Sanitary Commission publications would champion constitutional explanations for disease. Further, surgeons' preconceptions about soldier bodies would help to govern their attitudes toward their patients, especially when sorting alleged cases of malingering from those of genuine illness.

Another related traditional explanation for disease that addressed mental and physical health was hereditarianism. The theory purported to explain how traits were passed down from one generation to the next but, again, fostered more stereotypes than it provided helpful approaches to disease. In particular moments of susceptibility, such as conception, gestation, birth, or nursing, a parent could supposedly influence a child's personality, intellect, or constitution. Twins appeared to be living proof. Because they had experienced the same interactive moments as one another, they were more similar in personality and appearance than siblings born years apart. Such an understanding of disease causation left little room for physicians to consider the importance of preventative techniques. The only way that one might avoid passing along disease to one's child was to refrain from certain destructive behaviors, such as alcoholism or depression, during the sensitive moments of development. There was also an apparent gendered dimension to the supposition. Critical attention increasingly fell upon the mother, especially if she were lower class, who might be encouraged to forgo breastfeeding if she were considered sickly, mentally unstable, or depraved.[51]

Phrenology, a subset of hereditarianism, is perhaps the most infamous of nineteenth-century explanations for mental constitution. Like other hereditarian explanations, it excluded preventative possibilities and provided little guidance for treating mental health. Its pioneer Franz Joseph Gall mapped areas he termed "organs" of the brain to corresponding mental functions. In his charts of brain organization, he isolated such features as tenderness, arithmetic, wit, capacity for murder, or delight in colors. Gall postulated that the outer cranial structure could be measured to reflect the relative development of the brain faculties beneath. Thus, to the phrenologist, mental traits—such as intellectual capacity, personality, and morality—were innate, not learned. The concept starkly limited the possibilities for treating mental disorder. Phrenological journals generally just exhorted men and women to choose their mates carefully, as their union might have lasting consequences on their offspring.[52]

One of the more forward-thinking mental health theorists of the age was Dr. Isaac Ray, author of *Mental Hygiene*, who suggested a larger role for the patient in promoting wellness. Ray suggested that the concept of heredity might be substituted with the milder idea of predisposition. While a person with a mentally ill parent might have a predisposition to insanity, madness could be circumvented by a careful regimen geared toward increasing the health of the brain organ. Ray recommended exercise, appropriate diet, sleep, moderation in imbibing tea, coffee, or spirits, and, much to the delight of schoolchildren, he limited homework to allow time for recreation and hobbies. Parents were encouraged to provide moral instruction, which also could improve mental health. And yet habits and environment could only affect one's mental hygiene so much. Ray's work also cited differences among the races, insisting that a "native Australian" would never elevate to the intellectual stature of a "cultivated European," nor could the "unthinking multitude[s]" improve to the level of the "Bacons and Newtons of the world."[53]

Psychological theories would have limited effects on the lives of common soldiers in 1862, as most traditional doctors did not see promoting mental health as part of their purview.[54] Rather, these psychological theories reflected a tendency on the part of professional practitioners to associate mental health with class, as they generally believed the lower classes to be less intelligent and more prone to such defects as alcoholism. Both physical and mental health theories also suggested that it was not the domain of physicians to prevent disease, but rather that sickness at least partially depended upon the choices made by an individual. These attitudes would indeed shape interactions between soldiers and their surgeons at sick call and in hospital, as surgeons sometimes blamed undisciplined behavior in the ranks for soldier sickness and low morale.

Rather than the Civil War providing a moment for orthodox doctors to reassess their roles in patients' lives, the birth of professional associations shortly before the war only encouraged a re-entrenchment into the old norms. The 1847 American Medical Association, for instance, made sluggish progress toward establishing and enforcing standards but had fairly wide success at blocking alternative practitioners, such as homeopaths, from military service.[55] In the realm of asylum care, the repository of mental health care before the war, the 1844 Association of Medical Superintendents of American Institutions for the Insane, succeeded in blocking out unorthodox practitioners until the end of the nineteenth century.[56] These organizations arose to protect traditional physicians from the democratic attack on their status as experts. In 1862, some surgeons would correspondingly prove more concerned with power and rank than soldier care, while many also rejected the interference of middle-class reform workers within the military system.

Traditional American medicine would remain regressive during the war, but Europe was in the midst of a medical revolution. In France and Germany, a new enthusiasm for measuring—using stethoscopes, laryngoscopes, and opthalmoscopes—replaced the old adage that a physician's sense was more important than his measurements. Further, French scientist Xavier Bichat used autopsies and dissection to suggest that the body was composed of tissues, not humors. Pierre Louis followed up on this revelation by demonstrating that disease attacked and damaged solid tissues rather than the blood; therefore, there was no use in balancing the bodily fluids. In the 1840s and 1850s came more triumphs for scientific observation and measurements, this time in England. John Snow noticed the correlation between infected water and cholera, followed by William Budd, who discerned a similar effect with typhoid fever. Meanwhile in France, Louis Pasteur was beginning to observe particles in fermentation that would lead to his conception of the germ theory in the 1870s.[57] Despite the fact that a growing number of American doctors attended medical school abroad, these discoveries were in their early stages and would have limited impacts on treatment during the Civil War.

MIDDLE-CLASS REFORMERS AND ALTERNATIVE MEDICINE

The greatest challenge to the old medical identity in the Jacksonian period came from alternative healers, some of whom were also doctors by training. Like orthodox physicians, alternative practitioners presumed a special ability to supervise the health of the masses; however, many also advocated self-care and preventative medicine, enlarging the scope of traditional healing. Historians disagree on the extent to which the public preferred alternative healers, but the successful state-level deregulation of medical licensing suggests they enjoyed considerable sway. Historian Warner writes that alternative healers deployed "a radically democratic . . . rhetoric that had powerful resonances in American society," while Naomi Rogers argues that Jacksonian Americans chose their healers on a case-by-case basis.[58]

In the wake of the religious revival of the Second Great Awakening in the 1820s and 30s, moral reform bled over into the health arena. Health reformers advocated positive thinking, ethical behavior, nature-based treatments, and diet and exercise. This enthusiasm for grooming the body and mind was not altogether unlike modern self-help movements. As historian Frances Clarke has helped illuminate, the Northern middle class identified themselves as more adept than the rabble at self-discipline, morality, and coping with suffering. Those who could embrace but not overly indulge in the suffering endemic to antebellum life proved genteel, as did those who engaged in elaborate grieving rituals over the deaths of loved ones.[59] It followed that markers of low class included being less-equipped to prevent and manage disease and cope with its outcomes; therefore, it fell to the enlightened middle class to provide guidance. While orthodox physicians agreed with the idea that a lack of self-discipline could influence disease, they did not often publicly embrace the ethos of self-care, which would have rendered their services superfluous and aligned them too closely with alternative practitioners—consequences that ran counter to their project of professionalization.

The most influential "alternative" medical practitioners in the antebellum period were homeopaths. Homeopathy, invented by Samuel Hahnemann in Germany in 1810 and introduced into America in the 1830s, advanced several therapeutic philosophies: the law of the similar (administering medications that produced the symptoms of the diseases they were meant to treat) and the law of infinitesimals (using minute, undiluted quantities of these medicines). Diagnosis by a homeopath also required extensive patient interviews that could last hours.[60] The homeopathic project of reshaping medicine went beyond offering an alternative to what practitioners derisively termed "allopathic" or traditional medicine. Homeopaths wished to supplant the orthodox medicine they considered defective, igniting a competition with doctors that would rage from the 1830s through the 1860s.[61] By the advent of the Civil War, homeopaths had enjoyed considerable success in diverting healers from traditional medicine to their field. There were roughly 2,500 homeopathic healers in the United States (compared to 30,000 orthodox healers), five monthly journals, six homeopathic medical colleges, and a national homeopathic medical society.[62]

Homeopathy quickly blossomed in America because the medical field was already so diffuse. Indeed, the popularity of Thomsonian medicine, brainchild of self-taught herbalist Samuel Thomson, drew American followers as early as the first decade of the nineteenth century. Thomson stressed that understanding medicine was as simple as observing one's own body, that each person could and should act as his or her own doctor, and that botanical- and/or water-based treatments were superior to chemicals. And yet his concept of disease was not so far removed from humoral theory; his aim was to restore the body's "natural" heat, rather than fluid balance, often with hot peppers, steam, and purgatives.[63]

Homeopathic and Thomsonian medical schools advertised in the newspapers to attract students and to convince the court of public opinion of their superior methods. The Thomsonian Botanico-Medical College of Ohio in Cincinnati advertised in the *National ERA*: "This school believes in the unity of disease. . . . It rejects, for the healing of the sick, the lancet and every species of poisons, not only 'in the ordinary circumstances of their judicious application.'" It emphasized its endorsement of environmental cures, self-help, and prevention: "It uses the most active and innocent agents in the three-fold kingdom of nature . . . and devotes a large portion of its instructions to the Divine Art of Preserving Health, and Preventing nearly all the aches and ills that flesh is heir to."[64] These ideas coincided with popular Jacksonian ideals, winning significant American confidence before the Civil War.

Other popular movements transcended the narrow realm of disease to engage more broadly with social reformism. These movements would also touch soldiers, particularly Northerners, where reform had been more popular, and with whom the moral reformers of the U.S. Sanitary Commission interacted. Temperance, for instance, was a widespread antebellum crusade and would remain important in wartime given rampant alcohol consumption—both medicinal and recreational—in army camps. Many temperance advocates were women, as women were often the first victims of alcohol-induced violence; thus, temperance reform allowed women a role in prescribing behavior to improve health and social ills. One temperance leader, Rev. Sylvester Graham, asserted a more comprehensive health program called Grahamism. Graham advocated vegetarianism, consuming a coarsely ground wheat bread or crackers as one's main food staple, and moderation in drinking, eating, and sexual behavior.[65] Under Graham's tenets, the individual could exercise considerable control over his or her own well-being with proper self-discipline. Meanwhile hydropathy, which crossed the Atlantic Ocean from Germany in the 1840s, valued water cure, or soaking in healing waters at the sea or spas.[66] Water-cure enthusiasts, like Graham and other reformers, touted a particular diet— the renunciation of alcohol, tobacco, caffeine, and meat—and were ardent about their health care regimes. They ultimately believed that water, diet, and exercise could prevent and cure most sickness. While the financial ability to soak in spas distinguished the upper classes from the plebeians in the South, the practice remained more democratic in the North.[67]

On a related note, personal sanitation—bathing and using soap—had also gained popularity before the war and would, in turn, affect soldier cleanliness in 1862. Public debates over the connection between cleanliness and disease took wing right before the turn of the eighteenth century, and by the early 1800s some city dwellings were outfitted with baths and showers, and more Americans were using soap. Rural and lower-class Americans remained suspicious of full-body immersion much longer, viewing it as a potentially sinful pleasure, while the middle class more quickly came to view the practice as civil and genteel. Women again played a central role in the acceptance of sanitation as they became increasingly tasked with presiding over a clean and healthy home.[68] In any case, bathing and using soap were far more accepted practices during the Civil War than they had been in the past. Some common soldiers would make bathing a priority in their schedules, while others had to be forced to wash by their officers.

A related sanitation movement advocated by city-dwelling middle-class reformers was public health. Because Civil War armies would function like cities, public-health theories would gain even more relevance in 1862. Antebellum cities suffered frequent disease epidemics, such as yellow fever and cholera, and endured recurrent outbreaks of communicable diseases, such as measles, mumps, and scarlet fever. Public health reformers emphasized environment as a probable cause of the higher rates of illness, especially the omnipresent miasmas from sewage, air pollution, and trash. Public health outcries in British and U.S. cities in the 1840s and 1850s called for investigation into foul smells and public waters used for drinking, bathing, and washing. Public health boards and "smell committees" attempted to regulate air and water but with mixed results. While London experienced drastic improvements from its public health initiatives, citizens of Chicago, for instance, doubted the validity of the science underlying activism, because disease remained rampant.[69] Beyond miasma, public health officials also investigated the adverse effects of poverty on health and called for improved hygiene and well-balanced diets for the lower classes, as well as more attention to mental health. During the war, U.S. Sanitary Commission inspectors would take on the role of smell committees, sniffing out the sources of camp pollution and observing deficiencies in diet and morale.

Prewar reform also addressed mental health, and this growing concern would be reflected in wartime hospitals and the principles of the U.S. Sanitary Commission. The most widespread hypothesis was that attitude influenced physical health. If a sick person adopted a positive attitude, then he or she might enjoy a speedy recovery. If the patient, however, indulged in self-pity, then suffering could become unbearable, leading even to death. Both Confederate and Union hospitals frequently engaged in this line of reasoning with the soldiers under their care. Another prewar mental health initiative had to do with the small number of Americans who were seriously mentally ill, a population that would grow in the 1860s because of wartime trauma. New Englander Dorothea Dix led the charge to end the incarceration of the "insane" who had become unmanageable by their families or drifted beyond the fold of society. Appearing before legislatures in Northern and Southern states, Dix presented chilling tales of mentally unstable inmates locked in prison cages, underfed, and brutally punished. Her campaign successfully mobilized state funding for asylums across the nation.[70] While such reforms increased attention to mental health leading up to the war, health care workers lacked an adequate vocabulary to describe the full spectrum of mental problems. In 1862, the army Medical Departments would address only the most severe mental illnesses, but some middle-class reformers would display a more nuanced interest in soldier attitudes. Indeed, Dix herself would become U.S. wartime superintendent of female nurses.

Middle-class reformers thus considerably shaped antebellum ideas about disease causation, treatment, and mental health, wooing the underclasses with less invasive, nature-based treatments and the promotion of self-care. They would continue to affect health care during the war via the U.S. Sanitary Commission and other aid societies, writing newspaper articles and serving as nurses, doctors, and army officers. Their behavior-based approaches to health care would help clean up camps and often prove complimentary to soldier self-care, but their presumed superiority over the rank-and-file soldier would also become a source of tension.

To summarize the prewar state of American health care, future common soldiers were products of a complex and changing world. Their preference for home care, environmental explanations of disease, and taking responsibility for their own bodies would profoundly influence their behavior in 1862. But the war would not only foster cultural continuity; it would also bring paradigm shifts in common people's interactions with their environment and with health care workers. Whereas traditional doctors had once occupied limited roles in their patients' lives, as surgeons they became soldiers' primary point of entry into the military medical system, despite their chaotic understandings of disease and professional quarrels. Soldiers longed to be nursed by their loved ones but would now be attended by strangers in the most vulnerable moments of their lives.

War would also bring soldier behavior under increased scrutiny from the middle class, which was eager to exert its health programs over the masses and saw the health crisis of the Civil War as an ideal opportunity. While soldiers were grateful to such organizations as the Sanitary Commission, they would also exhibit a clear preference for care from each other, which came without judgment or agenda.

2

At War with Nature

Just a few days into first encampment, soldiers had to reexamine the presumption that those raised on the fresh air of country life had superior constitutions to the urban-bred. "Death invaded my camp," observed Capt. George Clark of Alabama, astonished by the swiftness of this transformation. Predictably, measles, mumps, small pox, scarlet fever, whooping cough, diphtheria, tuberculosis, and other communicable disease ravaged approximately half of new recruits, leaving the lucky survivors seasoned by the first transition to army life. Clark had to admit, he was confused: "Remarkable as it may seem, the stout country boys whom it may be supposed could stand all kinds of hardships, were the first to succumb while the city boys as a rule escaped."[1] It slowly dawned on soldiers that armies were cities—large cities. The Union Army of the Potomac would swell to be the second largest Southern metropolis after New Orleans, and the Army of Northern Virginia would reach over twice the size of Richmond. Those men who had been raised among urban crowds and filth were thus better suited to endure army conditions.

The transformation from rural to city landscape without sufficient infrastructures occurred right away, wherever armies marched. But from 1861 through 1862, soldiers began to observe an even more marked challenge to their prewar beliefs about seasoning. War had a leveling effect on bodies and disease locales. Southerners and Northerners alike were sick, not just on the Peninsula but in the Shenandoah Valley. Armies fouled water, dug entrenchments, contaminated soil with waste, and died in droves along with their animals, littering the landscape with bodies. This dismal environmental transformation would have been dangerous to health on its own, but soldiers were also supremely exposed to the elements, living almost exclusively outside with little protection. The men's written accounts were abuzz connecting environmental phenomena to the sudden proliferation of physical and mental ailments. They tried to make sense of change and continuity with their prewar ideas, growing anxious. They did not want to be one of the unlucky who succumbed to disease. "No one need shun death on the battlefield when such as he so young & full of strength & hope fall by disease," explained Lt. Charles B. Haydon of the 2nd Michigan.[2]

Many soldiers tried to dissuade loved ones from joining the ranks where they, too, might experience the terrible vulnerability of army life. "I kno it is the duty of every young man . . . to join the army and help to defend his country. But I wrote to John not to do it until he feels like he is able to stand a camp life. It takes a man who can shoulder his knapsack & musket and march 12 or 15 miles on a stretch as we have been doing for the last week. This is no place for the sick," explained Pvt. Lewis H. Bedingfield of Georgia to his parents, regarding his brother's impending enlistment.[3] It was only July 8, 1861, when he wrote those words, but Bedingfield was already engaged in the traumatic process of soldier seasoning, involving physical, psychological, and behavioral adaptations to the environment of war. Despite Lewis's fears, John and their third brother, Robert, did enlist in the autumn of 1861 to eventually participate in the Peninsula campaign. Unluckily, it would be Lewis who fell, mortally wounded at Gaines's Mill on June 27, 1862, expiring July 3 in a Richmond hospital. Bob would become sick with dysentery that same June, and John would attend to both brothers in their misery—Lewis in Richmond before he died and Bob in Staunton.[4] Unlike his brothers who were privates, John enjoyed the flexibility of being a commissioned officer—a first lieutenant—and so could briefly leave the ranks to oversee their health care.

Before soldiers could learn to protect themselves from the environment of war, they had to understand it. When they were not engaged in combat (which was most of the time), men, such as the Bedingfields, would devote inordinate amounts of time to observing the connections between their bodies and nature. They believed their lives depended on acquiring such knowledge, and in many cases they were correct. In other cases, such as Lewis's, death was simply unavoidable.

THE CAMPAIGNS AND ENVIRONMENTAL EXPOSURE

Before engaging with the soldiers' environmental descriptions of health, the two campaigns in which they were involved require some introduction. What the particular environments entailed, when and where the soldiers moved, and the logistical circumstances under which they operated all influenced their degree of exposure. While the net effect would be that soldiers were very ill and demoralized in both locations, there were different specifics at play.

The 1862 Shenandoah Valley campaign and the preceding Romney campaign in January presented a challenging combination of mountainous terrain and variable weather, constant movement, and logistical snafu. The geographic space of the Valley encompasses the Shenandoah River watershed, extending roughly southwest from the Potomac River to Lexington for about 140 miles. The Alleghenies punctuate the western border while the Blue Ridge Mountains mark the east, facing each other like chess pieces across a great, crisscrossing board of farms. The Shenandoah River flows north, lending itself to peculiar terminology: the Northern region is the Lower Valley and the Southern portion the Upper Valley. Likewise, to go "up" the Valley is to go south and to go "down" the Valley is to venture north. Traversing the Valley landscape was a laborious undertaking during the Civil War. It did not just mean plodding on the macadamized Valley Turnpike, one of the best roads in the Confederacy. In reality, even the Turnpike was hard and unforgiving on infantry feet when it froze or when traversed by the improperly shod. But soldering in the Valley necessarily meant braving the mountains, the largest of which, Massanutten, stands 2,900 feet tall near Harrisonburg with only one passable gap. The Alleghenies and Blue Ridge Mountains also possessed few passages, each narrow, requiring treacherous climbs with heavy gear.[5] Because of the varied terrain, the Valley attracted formidable weather — alternating snow, rain, wind, and ice.

Despite its natural challenges and its transformation to active campaign site during the war, the idea of the Valley as salubrious would be difficult for soldiers to shake. Soldiers in both gray and blue frequently marveled at the region's beauty. "I looked upon this great handiwork of Creation and wondered if an atheist could look upon this and say there is no God," wrote Stonewall Brigade hospital steward John S. Apperson. Lt. Col. David H. Strother, a Virginia-born Yankee, concurred: "The sight of this beautiful valley, its rural wealth and improvements, seemed to have softened the hearts of officers and men."[6] Pvt. Thomas Ellis, an infantryman in the 111th Pennsylvania, could lament his disease environment and still praise the Valley's majestic scenery in one breath: "We had to march 2 days through a verry hard rain and then lay down in wet clothes on the wet cold ground. it has caused a great deal of sickness in our camps nearly all the soldiers are troubled with the dioreah. The Valley of the Shaunandoah is one of the finest that I have ever seen in all my travels. . . . I think that this must be a very healthy country. Though very warm," he added with little concern over his apparent contradiction.[7]

While most troops had settled into winter quarters by early 1862, Maj. Gen. Thomas "Stonewall" Jackson, promoted to command the Valley District in November of 1861, was eager to seize the initiative gained by the Confederate victory at First Manassas and make something active of traditional winter lethargy. In December, Jackson refused to grant furloughs, a miscalculation of his men's fortitude that would later lead to tremendous disciplinary strife, and instead trained his men at Winchester, waiting for reinforcements to fulfill his proposed plan to move along the Baltimore and Ohio Railroad (B&O) and drive out the enemy from northwestern Virginia. The nearby Union generals in the Valley, Maj. Gen. Nathaniel P. Banks and Brig. Gen. William S. Rosecrans, were stymied by General-in-Chief George B. McClellan's refusal to take seriously their proposals to march up the Valley on Winchester, allowing Jackson to dictate winter events. McClellan instead wintered Banks and his 16,000 near Frederick, Maryland, while Brig. Gen. William Rosecrans's 22,000 splayed out along the B&O.[8]

Jackson's Romney campaign began when the general marched his nearly 11,000 men from Winchester to Bath on January 1, 1862, an unseasonably warm day that portended a sudden freeze. The campaign was hardly a pleasant alternative to winter camp, with long, slow marches in snow, sleet, and winds. The Romney Pike was frozen solid, and the Rebels lacked food and blankets and shivered in the zero-degree days. By the time Jackson made it to Bath on January 4 and Romney on January 14, both had been abandoned, yielding a bounty of Federal supplies, and yet the Confederates were forced to bivouac in lice-ridden buildings and frigid open fields. Having cleared the area of the enemy, Jackson took only his Stonewall Brigade back up to Winchester, leaving behind Brig. Gen. William W. Loring's three brigades to hold the ground in the dead of winter.[9] Loring's officers, enraged by what they viewed as unnecessary suffering, sickness, and demoralization in their ranks, signed a petition asking to be removed to Winchester, engendering a command dispute that almost resulted in Jackson's resignation.[10]

By the time Confederate authorities ordered Loring's forces back to headquarters at Winchester, Jackson had gained a reputation for cruelty, exposing his men to the bitter cold for what was deemed a fruitless campaign. Indeed, by February, all the ground that the general had gained in the Romney campaign had fallen to Federals. That month compounded Confederate misery with severe rains, and March dawned with extremely variable weather, one day fine and the next cold, drizzly, or snowy. Winchester ballooned into a ghastly spectacle of the sick.[11]

In March, Jackson was instructed to pin down in the lower Valley both Banks's 20,000, who had plans to return to the Washington vicinity, and the 8,000 Federals in the Allegheny Mountains under Maj. Gen. John C. Frémont, Rosecrans's replacement and head of the newly formed Mountain Department. Frémont would soon grow horrified at his inability to provide supplies, food, and medical necessities for his army, but he was not the first Confederate target: the division Banks had left to defend the lower Valley under Brig. Gen. James Shields was. Jackson threw a small force against Shields at Kernstown on March 23, which ended in disorderly Confederate retreat up the Valley. Jackson's tactical loss was a strategic gain, however, as Banks's full force doubled back to the Valley to confront the Rebels. Given Jackson's threat, President Abraham Lincoln kept at his disposal Maj. Gen. Irvin McDowell's 40,000 at Fredericksburg rather than allotting them to Maj. Gen. George B. McClellan's campaign to take Richmond.[12] Union command in the Valley region was thus fragmented, compounded by the fact that on March 11 Lincoln had demoted McClellan from general-in-chief to mere commanding general of the Army of the Potomac because of persistent disputes. It would prove difficult to correct logistical deficiencies in the leadership void that followed.[13] Historian Carmen B. Grayson has given evidence that even U.S. quartermaster general Montgomery C. Meigs was preoccupied by providing strategic advice to Secretary of War Edwin M. Stanton and Lincoln rather than attending to his own job during the Shenandoah Valley and Peninsula campaigns.[14]

Banks marched on Harrisonburg, occupying it on April 25, while Jackson withdrew to Swift Run Gap, where he combined with Brig. Gen. Edward Johnson's division, tricking Banks into believing that the Confederates had quit the Valley altogether. Therefore, when Lincoln ordered Banks to move to Strasburg and Shields to join McDowell's troops, Jackson was free to attack. Attack he did. On May 8 at McDowell, Jackson's reinforced command fired upon a fragment of Frémont's army under Brig. Gen. Robert H. Milroy, who had come from the Alleghenies to threaten Jackson's supply depot at Staunton. Tactically the Union army inflicted heavier casualties but was forced to withdraw, yielding the strategic gain to Jackson, as he no longer faced a threat from the Alleghenies. Jackson then turned his attention to Banks at Strasburg, and Banks, sensing danger, detached the U.S. 1st Maryland Infantry to meet Jackson at Front Royal. On May 23, the Union regiment was overrun by the more than 17,000 under Jackson's command and surrendered. Banks was forced to

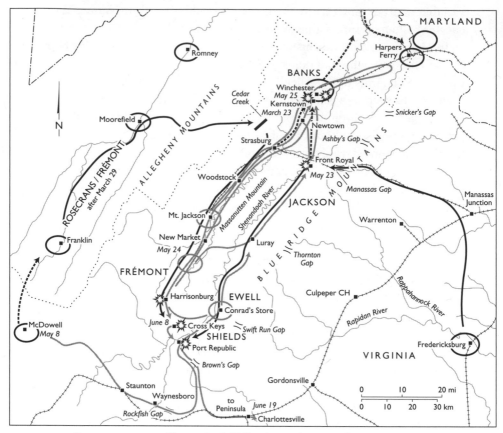

MARYLAND

Romney

Harpers
Ferry

BANKS

Winchester
May 25
Kernstown
March 23

*Cedar
Creek*

Snicker's Gap

Moorefield

Newtown

Strasburg

Ashby's Gap

ROSECRANS / FRÉMONT
after March 29

Woodstock

Front Royal

May 23

Manassas Gap

Manassas
Junction

JACKSON

Mt. Jackson

Warrenton

Franklin

New Market

May 24

Luray

*Thornton
Gap*

FRÉMONT

Culpeper CH

EWELL

Harrisonburg

Conrad's Store

June 8

Cross Keys

Swift Run Gap

McDowell
May 8

SHIELDS

Port Republic

Fredericksburg

VIRGINIA

Brown's Gap

Staunton

Gordonsville

Waynesboro

0   10   20 mi

Rockfish Gap

to
Peninsula *June 19*

0   10   20   30 km

Charlottesville

*Troop movements, Shenandoah Valley Campaign, March 23–June 9, 1862
(based on maps by Hal Jespersen, www.cwmaps.com)*

retreat toward Winchester, where the battle of First Winchester occurred on May 25, engaging the full force of Rebels and only 6,500 Federals—another Jackson victory—resulting in Banks withdrawing across the Potomac River. Jackson, however, did not pursue Banks because his men were spent by their hard marching.[15]

Still, Jackson did not spare his men for long. He spurred them on to Harpers Ferry, compelling Lincoln to divert McDowell's command from Fredericksburg to the Valley just as McDowell was about to descend upon the Rebel capital from above, hampering the Peninsula campaign. Lincoln hoped to intercept Jackson before he moved up the Valley on the Pike, and so ordered Frémont to Harrisonburg. Frémont's men were hideously encumbered by lack of food and bad weather, which resulted in impassable roads and impenetrable mountain gaps. Instead, Frémont would march through the Alleghenies toward Strasburg, while McDowell was supposed to threaten Strasburg from Front Royal. Weather prevented McDowell from fulfilling his role, and the Confederates escaped through Strasburg. Rain then delayed Shields's men from assisting, leaving only Frémont to pursue Jackson. After six days of exhausting chase, two confrontations between Frémont and Jackson occurred at Cross Keys on June 8 and Port Republic on June 9. The twin U.S. losses effectively ended the campaign, and Banks and Shields evacuated the Valley. The Shenandoah Valley campaign from March to mid-June had become the hike of a lifetime; by its end, many of Jackson's foot soldiers had marched approximately 650 miles. The fragmented Union armies had marched less but had gravely suffered from the trying weather and lack of supplies. By mid-June, Jackson received a summons from new Army of Northern Virginia commander Robert E. Lee to join the campaign to protect the Confederate capital.[16] By the time Jackson reached Lee, he and his men could scarcely function from exhaustion.

Contemporary reports revealed the Valley campaign to have been sickly, but not nearly as destructive to health as the soldiers' accounts would reveal. In April 1862, the U.S. Sanitary Commission reported to the *Chicago Tribune* that in the Valley area there were 162 sick men for every thousand, versus sixty-three to every thousand in the Army of the Potomac.[17] This report (while low) confirms that the Valley was indeed sicklier than the Peninsula in spring, while the Peninsula would prove unhealthier in summer. Before General Rosecrans was relocated, he noted in March, "The proportion of sick and absent in the Districts of the Big Sandy and the Gap may be presumed to be about 20 per cent. Whence it appears that from the total strength given in this report it will be fair to deduct 20 to 25 per cent. in order to obtain the number fit for duty."[18] Confederate records are less complete, but regimental medical reports in the Valley reveal that for many regiments there were nearly as many cases of sickness as men.[19] Jackson's troops had the worst fortunes—they had endured hard marching during the most taxing Valley weather and were now bound for the Peninsula, a mosquito-dense quagmire in summer.

The Peninsula campaign was similarly challenging when it came to weather (though slightly less variable than the Valley), but it differed in that its slow pace led to more camp filth and resultant diarrhea and typhoid, while its swampy terrain produced more malaria. The fact the campaign dragged on well into the summer and involved much larger armies meant that it would yield more sickness overall than the Shenandoah Valley campaign. The fate of the campaign was also indelibly intertwined with events in the Valley. Jackson's offensive diverted Union resources, while the fractured Union command hampered both campaigns. Yet even aside from these problems, McClellan's pursuit of Richmond and Confederate general Joseph E. Johnston's defense of the capital proved a sluggish endeavor marked by slow movement, siege, and retreat.

After breaking winter camp in March, Union soldiers set sail on the Potomac River and down the Chesapeake Bay to the tip of the Virginia Peninsula at Fort Monroe. The Virginia Peninsula is the finger of land jutting out into the bay flanked by the York and James Rivers. The Chickahominy River slices through the center of the Peninsula, generating swampy terrain that is extremely susceptible to flooding and did so frequently that year. Soldiers did not have high hopes for their health in such miasmatic terrain, and their 1862 descriptions confirmed this bias. A Union cavalry officer remembered, "The forests between the York and the James rivers were filled with tangled thickets and unapproachable morasses. The tributaries of the rivers, mostly deep, crooked and sluggish, became more tortuous as they approach their confluence, and the expanse of floods is converted by evaporation into their stagnant swamps. A heavy rain in a few hours rendered these streams formidable obstacles. Above this dismal landscape the fierce rays of the sun were interrupted only at night, or by deluges of rain, so that men and animals were alternately scorched and drenched."[20] Spring of 1862 was cold, with days that did not break free from the thirties; however, temperatures by the end of April crept into the forties and fifties. Spring on the Peninsula was far superior to the heat, humidity, and insects that summer would bring.[21]

Instead of a quick fight, the newly arrived Union troops were treated to McClellan's specialty: waiting. He initiated a siege at Yorktown on April 5, fearing that the enemy outnumbered him. In reality, McClellan's army of

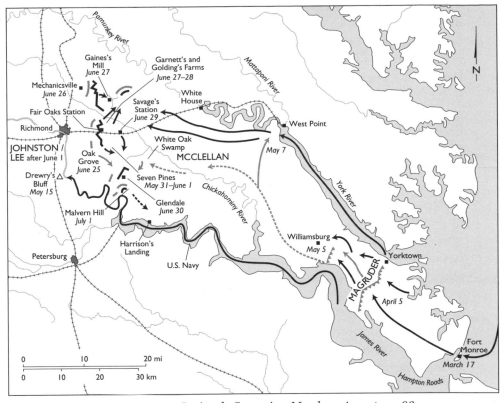

Troop movements, Peninsula Campaign, March 17–August 15, 1862
(based on maps by Hal Jespersen, www.cwmaps.com)

over 120,000 was facing just John Magruder's 12,000. The siege dragged on for a month, giving commanding Confederate general Johnston time to arrive with his army. The Confederates withdrew on May 3 into a slow retreat, and the rainy battle of Williamsburg on May 5 was a clash of the Confederate rearguard (eventually amounting to 32,000) against 41,000 Federals. Johnston's army then continued its withdrawal toward Richmond, while the Union gave slow chase. McClellan eventually crossed the Chickahominy River, the last real impediment to the Confederate capital, only to hunker down upon its swampy banks, split three corps on the Northern side and two on the Southern. May remained stormy, washing out roads and swelling the river, so McClellan delayed again, building bridges and requesting reinforcements, despite outnumbering Johnston by perhaps 40,000. The standoff finally came to an end when Johnston, under pressure from Richmond, broke the stalemate. On May 31 to June 1, he initiated the battle of Fair Oaks or Seven Pines, which was inconclusive other than Johnston's severe wounding, taking him out of the field.[22]

President Davis, who had come to observe the battle, placed Robert E. Lee in charge the following day. Lee took nearly a month to discipline and build up his newly christened Army of Northern Virginia (90,000 strong). He further planned a new offensive to repulse the enemy from Richmond, ordering Jackson to join him and cavalry general J. E. B. Stuart to reconnoiter around the Army of the Potomac, while McClellan ploddingly moved his guns closer to Richmond. On June 25, Lee inaugurated the Seven Days battles at Oak Grove, north of the Chickahominy, involving relatively few units and not bringing conclusive results.[23] June 26 saw another confrontation at Mechanicsville/Beaver Dam Creek with larger forces (14,000–15,000 per side), a tactical victory for the Union, but McClellan fell back to Gaines's Mill. A significant battle (36,000–57,000 engaged per side) followed at Gaines's Mill on June 27 with Confederate victory but only after a very poor performance from the exhausted Jackson and his men. Meanwhile, fights broke out at Garnett's and Golding's Farms among several divisions on June 27–28. On June 29, as the Union army withdrew toward the James River, Lee struck its rearguard near Savage's Station, while Jackson was delayed north of the Chickahominy. The Federals abandoned supplies and 2,500 sick and wounded to retire through White Oak Swamp. Engagements ensued at White Oak Swamp and Glendale (June 30), where McClellan was able to prevent Lee from blocking his retreat, at least in part because of deficient Confederate execution. Jackson, for one, had spent the better part of the fight asleep under a tree. By July 1, McClellan established a strong position at Malvern Hill, which Lee vigorously but unsuccessfully assaulted. Despite Union victory, McClellan completed his retreat to Harrison's Landing on the James River, yielding a strategic Confederate win. The Peninsula campaign was over.[24]

The summer weather had been punishing. Half of the June days were marked by heaving rains, and some of the sultrier days crested at ninety-two degrees. July was even more stifling. During at least twenty-two of the days, temperatures soared from eighty to ninety-five degrees, and August brought additional withering heat: twenty-four days of heat that dangled in the upper eighties to mid-nineties.[25] Contemporary sick reports, while vast underestimates, portrayed change over time. By June on the Peninsula, an estimated twenty-four percent of over 100,000 Federal troops were listed as no longer fit for duty; by July, twenty-nine percent were reported as ailing.[26] As early as March 1862, the Army of Northern Virginia's 49,394 troops had suffered approximately 149,148 cases of illness, and this number rose dramatically throughout the summer. Many of the cases on both sides were diarrhea or dysentery, which carried a ten percent mortality rate.[27] The spikes in illness coincided with long encampments, such as at the siege at Yorktown, the standoff at the Chickahominy River in May through June, and the Army of the Potomac's July and August sojourn at Harrison's Landing, which featured a ghastly diarrhea epidemic. The Federals' plummeting health played a factor in McClellan's decision to quit Harrison's Landing in mid-August. Lee felt similarly: "I think the health as well as discipline of the Army will be benefited by a change to the Country from the town & the city itself receive a more healthy atmosphere," he wrote to President Davis.[28]

When laid out together, the action involved in the two campaigns appears considerable, but the individual engagements reveal that most soldiers were seldom engaged in combat (excluding Stonewall Jackson's troops). Men, in fact, spent the majority of their time concerned with the other enemy that had dictated movement and, to their thinking, caused staggering sickness and despondency in the ranks. That enemy was environment—the weather, climate, seasons, terrain features, flora, and fauna that they could not avoid, exposed as they were by lack of supplies, a pace too quick in the Valley to secure proper protection and too slow on the Peninsula to avoid befouled soil and water, and swarms of disease-bearing insects.

"THIS IS NO PLACE FOR THE SICK"

If one environmental theme emerged from the two campaigns, it was rain. "Rain was the greatest discomfort a soldier could have; it was more uncomfortable than the severest cold with clear weather," remembered Pvt. Carlton McCarthy of Virginia, though his days of lying outside with the Army of Northern Virginia were long since past.[29] Worse than its discomfort, rain put men on "the sick list," or so 3rd Vermont Infantryman Pvt. George Q. French suspected.[30] Precipitation was the most commonly cited cause of disease in 1862, and official Union medical records confirm that the spike in wet, cold weather in the Shenandoah Valley corresponded to increased rates of sickness.[31] One Pennsylvania cavalryman stationed in the Valley explained the process by which rain led to sickness in more detail: "There is nothing in our mode of life to injure our health, but exposure to all kinds of weather. Sometimes we have to stay out all night, and the ground is now so muddy that we cannot walk fast without getting our feet wet, and consequently cold."[32] A Virginian on the Peninsula similarly wrote that "service on the Peninsula" was "arduous and disagreeable; in the muddy trenches, or back in the woods, lying on the rain-soaked ground, or marching along the cut-up and muddy roads, was trying indeed, and caused no little sickness among the troops."[33] Though spring rains were familiar to Virginians, they appeared just as hampered by the effects as did outsiders.

It was difficult to decide in which scenario rain was a worse tormentor, when trying to achieve a night's rest or when trekking through the viscous mud with full gear. In either case, rain dampened soldiers' spirits. Camping in March, a Stonewall Brigade man's morale sank: "Rain all night. Bed clothes wet. Cold and Cheerless day. Felt very unhappy, very sad, and very uncomfortable." It only got worse for him in April: "It soon commenced raining and for three days it has hailed and rained and snowed in the most unaccountable manner. Our encampment is worse than any barnyard for in many places there seems no bottom." As a consequence, he lapsed into inaction: "I laid in bed a long while rather than expose myself to the bitter dawn and cold. My heart was very sad. Our great discomfort and our cause weighed down upon me."[34] Strikingly, the description was written by a major. Officers had better access to supplies and shelter, and it was their job to promote morale in the ranks. When officer motivation disintegrated, so too did the structural sources of encouragement for enlisted men. Pvt. Fraiser Rosenkrans of the 44th New York Infantry stationed near the Chickahominy River proved in need of cheering. He suffered from fever and headache after marching fifteen miles by noon "in the rain with the mud from four to ten inches in depth." After ten days of illness, he pondered his own mortality: "I begin to realize that man is as grass and his days as the flower of grass. A death here seems to make but little impression on our minds."[35] Colonel Strother felt vocal concern for his men: "Warm rain. Have suffered all day with dullness and discouragement arising doubt-less from physical exhaustion. The wet weather and the fact of our retreat to this place seem to have cowed and irritated everybody."[36] Across the muddy, sodden expanse of Virginia, enlisted men and even their officers appeared in danger of giving up though they had scarcely seen combat.

Soldiers were often very precise in linking rain to ague (which caused chills, fever, and sweating), malaria and typhoid (which produced fever, sore throat, diarrhea, fatigue, and pain), rheumatism (aches and pains), and, most commonly, diarrhea and dysentery (inflammation of the intes-tine with severe and often bloody diarrhea). "The Friday and Saturday be-fore, it rained very hard; my blankets, boots, and everything I had got wet. My throat troubled me considerably," recorded Pvt. Robert Carter from the Peninsula.[37] Officers, such as Capt. Henry Newton Comey, were convinced that the persistent "cold" rain took "its toll, as many of the men came down with chills and fever."[38] Some believed that if only the rain would cease, their ailments would improve. A New York Zouave wrote, "I have had quite a cold for about two weeks past, and I cough at night—I suppose that it will wear off as soon as warm weather sets in. There have been a number of men discharged already on account of disability—camp-life beginning to tell on them."[39] Pvts. James T. Miller, John C. Ellis, and Irvin Fox—all Union soldiers in the Valley—blamed the wet conditions for rampant di-arrhea. Miller felt the "hard watter" and "marching and sleeping in the rain" made "one half of our regiment sick with the dysentery," while Fox eschewed his surgeon's remedy of quinine for his diarrhea, which he found "rather poor medicine for soldiers who have to sleep on the damp ground & are exposed to nearly every rain storm."[40] Fox's analysis suggested that what men craved was better protection from the elements—a supply problem—rather than medicine. Others still complained of chill-induced cramps and spasms that made them too exhausted to be effective soldiers. Lt. Charles B. Haydon of the 2nd Michigan Infantry explained, "I had, as well as most of the men, by this time become so chilled by the rain & exhausted by our exertions to arrive on the field in time that our legs & arms were cramping so that we could scarcely use them." Haydon "was never nearer dead with cold & hunger. . . . I warmed and dried myself the best I could which was not very well as it rained in torrents, till midnight."[41]

Though rain was the most frequently recorded environmental threat to health, it was not the only dreaded weather condition; heat also attacked mental and physical health. Brig. Gen. Philip Kearny, a frequent critic of McClellan's slow advance on the Peninsula, worried in April, "I only fear, lest the approaching warm weather will decimate our army, if not, break it up with sickness."[42] He was correct to dread the warmer months. On May 2, a Pennsylvanian wrote his wife from the Peninsula that "the sun comes down to us poor mortals with more force than I ever felt before it is hot enough to day to cook eggs in its power, my head suffers sorely with the heat. . . . I wish [McClellan] might drive the reble army to hell so as to let us out of the swamp."[43] And Private McCarthy remembered that the sun in combination with the dust made for grueling marches: "In summer time, the dust, combined with the heat, caused great suffering. The nostrils of the men, filled with dust, became dry and feverish, and even the throat did not escape. The 'grit' was felt between the teeth, and the eyes were rendered almost useless."[44] Besides inciting general suffering, heat could literally sicken or kill, as Confederate James Huffman concluded. "On the 8th [of July], we moved back to White Oak Swamp, about ten miles. Here the smell was almost unendurable and the sun so extremely hot that men fell in the ranks, exhausted or from sunstroke."[45]

Rev. A. M. Stewart, who marched with the Army of the Potomac, was able to come to a more nuanced understanding of the effects of heat on health in his memoirs. "Hot weather is not necessarily unhealthy; yet in this oppressive heat, and under our conditions of camp life, it proves no easy matter for the multitudes who come here greatly debilitated, and with the seeds of disease contracted in the marshes of the Chickahominy, to become speedily restored to vigor."[46] Thus, Stewart believed after the war that it was not simply weather but the conditions of soldering that led to illness. Those same conditions could cause demoralization in even the most determined soldier. Lieutenant Haydon wrote that on May 13, it had grown so hot that his unit was ordered to halt by the Medical Department. Relief quickly gave way to suffering. "After all that is said abt toilsome marches they are not so bad as lying hour after hour on the bare ground, just plowed, in a roasting sun without tree or bush for shelter. One loses all patience & suffers both in body & mind."[47] Despite the best intentions of the medical officer in charge, resting in the heat was a punishment worse than marching.

Based on prewar notions about the South as a toxic disease climate, subject to dangerous seasonal shifts, soldiers also loquaciously examined these topics. The men grew most concerned with climate—typically de-scribed as the prevailing temperature, winds, and weather of an area—in the late spring and summer, which was associated with an increase in fevers and diarrhea. Their prewar biases against the Peninsula also meant that more attention was given to climate there than in the Valley. Capt. William Thompson Lusk, a soldier of more means than enlisted men, wrote home, "My dear Mother: My experience in South Carolina has not specially fitted me to resist climatic influences [on the Peninsula]. It will be incalculable advantage to me if I can get North three or four weeks this summer."[48] Lusk had probably ventured north to escape sickness in the past and hoped to secure leave for a similar purpose that summer. Other soldiers were surprised by their own resilience, finding that popular lore about the Peninsula did not always ring true. Sgt. Shepard G. Pryor recorded, "Wee are getting along verry well here now, standing the hardships of this climate much better than I expected," though Pryor noted this in February on the Peninsula, well before the onset of summer ailments.[49] The majority of soldiers, however, remained concerned about the potential adverse effects of the Southern climate on the human body. As Pvt. Robert G. Carter wrote home, "I feel very sad, more so than I ever did before, for I feel as though I should never see all my brothers again. . . . To lose either by sickness or wounds I know it would be a crushing blow to me. . . . They are coming from a northern climate into a much warmer and unhealthy one; the heat and water will affect them, I know."[50] And Lieutenant Haydon compared the soldier experience to the antebellum problem of migration: "This lying on the ground all the time is similar in its effect & the diseases it produces to those caused by moving into a new country. In the latter case the air is more impregnated with disease but the exposure is less."[51] On the whole, soldiers believed escalating sick tolls confirmed the dangers inherent in the Southern climate.

Considering their farming roots, many men continued to refer to cycles of sickness based on the seasons. In a letter to his mother and sisters in early August, Sgt. Oscar Ladley of the 75th Ohio wrote, "The sickly season is upon us and there will be a good deal of it I am afraid."[52] Pvt. William C. McClellan of Alabama noted that "in the summer season the Water is Warm and filthy."[53] A soldier from the 16th Massachusetts believed the seasons of Virginia had left a permanent stain upon his well-being, though he had finally recovered from a bout of illness that had kept him from his regiment for over a year. "I am here once more—not, alas! Long to remain; for exposure to the Virginia summer's heat and winter's cold, together with privations and hardships necessarily incident to campaigns such as ours have been, these have done their work, and for years I can scarcely hope to be as well in the future as I have been in the past."[54] This soldier may have, in fact, been hoping for another sojourn from the ranks—a potential malingerer. Nevertheless his fears were corroborated by his experience.

Early in 1862, some Confederates believed that Virginia's unpredictable seasons might significantly shape the time and place of the imminent

Federal campaign. Pvt. David Watson of the 53rd Virginia wrote, "I have never believed the [Yankee] expedition was intended for any place but some Southern port from the fact that the Yankees must know that the weather is too uncertain here at this season fir them to undertake any operation."[55] Though McClellan carried on his Peninsula campaign in spite of the sickly season, his troops certainly suffered from its effects. What soldiers like Watson learned was that war required that men endure environmental exposure that would have been considered unacceptable in peacetime.

Aside from weather, climate, and seasons, soldiers also scrutinized local terrain for causes of sickness and demoralization. In a rare depiction of soldiers at war with nature rather than their human enemy, a drawing appearing on January 18 in *Harper's Weekly* showed Union soldiers clawing their way through a Virginia forest that appeared to fight back.[56] The Peninsula and Valley each had its share of challenging terrain, made worse by the weather. The Shenandoah Valley campaign forced men to traverse rocky mountain passes and frigid roads, testing the limits of human endurance. Pvt. William F. Brand in the 5th Virginia was a participant in Stonewall Jackson's January Romney expedition. He was certain that marching through the Valley's challenging terrain in the snow would ravage the ranks, as horses and men slipped on roads that were "a perfect cake of ice." He wrote home, "We are now in 25 miles of Winchester & are campt on the Rumney road. I do not know what the Gen. intentions are if we are kept in this mountainous Country long one fourth of the army will be in the hospital for thare are loads going every day five of our Com has gone to the hospital & as many are sick in Camp."[57] On the Peninsula, swampland was unpleasant to wade through, but the rivers, particularly flooded rivers, created an obstacle to movement and immense frustration from General McClellan at the top down into the ranks of common soldiers. Confederate Pvt. Robert T. Hubard remarked that the Peninsula "country is very flat and much of the surface is submerged during a long, rainy season."[58] Traipsing through such sodden terrain ensured the men would remain wet, which prompted Union Surgeon Alfred L. Castleman to write, "Sickness among the troops rapidly increasing. Remittent fever, diarrhoea, and dysentery prevail. We are encamped in low, wet ground, and the heavy rains keep much of it overflowed. I fear that if we remain here long we shall lose many men by sickness."[59]

In a similar vein, Pvt. John O'Farrell, camped seven miles from Richmond in June, wrote, "Our camp is in a miserable place and has been named 'Quicksand.'"[60] Mud was indeed the most common grievance regarding terrain during both rain-drenched campaigns, and perhaps one

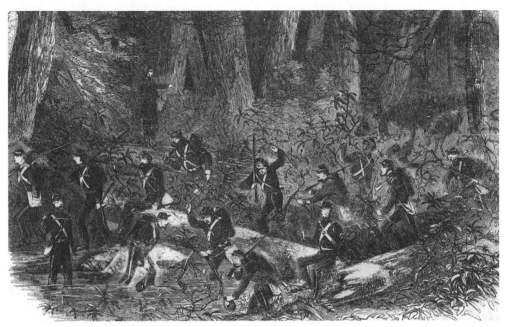

"The War in Virginia—A Reconnaissance in a Laurel Brake"
(Harper's Weekly, *January 18, 1862*)

of the most storied soldier complaints of the war. Rev. Joseph H. Twichell dreamed of constructing a "regimental arc" to navigate the "floating sea of mud" of his camp. "The porous, spongy, soil of the country is completely dissolved to an indefinite depth," he lamented.[61] Captain Clark nearly drowned in mud near Richmond. "I remember in going back to Richmond in the dark, that I stepped into quicksand and sank up to my shoulder. It was fortunate for me that two or three of my boys got hold of me in time to pull me out before I sank any further."[62] Some of the men believed this exposure to wet mud made them ill, but the most immediate effect of mud was to diminish morale. Private Carter of Massachusetts wistfully pondered, "There was hardly a man who did not tumble headlong [into mud] at least once. They looked as little like human beings as any men I ever saw. All were drenched with rain to the skin & cased with mud to the waist at least."[63] Union Quartermaster William G. Le Duc on the Peninsula wrote that in the worst of the mud, it was every man for himself. Bogged down in two feet of "adhesive mud," chaos ensued. "The tangle and confusion were indescribable, and there was almost a panic among the drivers. . . . The road, on each side, was occupied by lines of wet, bedraggled soldiers, marching doggedly through the mud. I appealed to them to help [unload an overloaded ambulance] . . . but they were wet, muddy, and miserable, and would not stop."[64] Le Duc could hardly blame the poor fellows; he too was despondent.

Another major environmental factor, most commonly feared by soldiers on the Peninsula, was miasma. Swamps looked and smelled threatening, and thus common sense seemed to substantiate the miasma theory, especially to those who had never seen a swamp until the war. Soldiers most often linked miasma to malaria and other fevers, and they were not so far afield of the truth given that mosquitoes were attracted to standing water and damp conditions. Descriptions captured large swamps "reeking with malaria," which were, in fact, teeming with malaria-bearing mosquitoes.[65] Though General McClellan was very popular with his men in 1862, some of them disparaged his notoriously slow advance through the swamps in their memoirs. Capt. Samuel A. Craig remembered that the general "was much criticised for stopping before Yorktown, it being alleged he could have driven out the force there a first, if he had the push. I remember too, letters criticising this halt by Dr. A. P. Heichhold, our regimental surgeon, to our home papers. . . . Many of our company got swamp fever, and there was much sickness, with wet mucky weather."[66] Some Confederates gleefully anticipated the destruction the Peninsula miasmas would wreck upon their enemies, such as Pvt. John Y. Beall of the 2nd Virginia. "McClellan now is encamped on the hills and bluffs of the James, his left on the river, his right on the swamps of the Chickahominy. This country is extremely unhealthy, being exposed to the malarious and miasmatic winds which every day blow between the rivers. Fever and ague and cholera, especially abound in this part of the world, and yellow-fever has always loved it. His army, with its strength shattered by fatigue, hunger, excitement, and dispirited by defeat, must fall by thousands before fevers and sickness."[67] Beall incorrectly assumed that his own army would be less vulnerable, given their prewar seasoning. Confederates soon learned otherwise; for instance, Lt. Campbell Brown of the 3rd Tennessee noted, "The loss of our Divn in killed & wounded was 985—mostly at Cold Harbor [Gaines's Mill]. But the seeds of disease sown by the malaria of the swamps carried off a good many more."[68]

Some soldiers feared that foul smells from the bodies of the dead might also transmit miasmatic disease, a supposition confirmed by many contemporary physicians. Private Carter wrote that "when we first came [to the Peninsula] a great number of cattle, sheep, hogs &c were killed all about the woods & fields, the offal of which with dead mules & horses as well as the necessary accumulations of filth abt large camps all combine to render the air unwholesome & sometimes at night & m'g the stench is almost insupportable." This was compounded by "the low marshy nature of the ground, the heavy rains & hot sultry days which invariably follow. There is not much sickness yet but it can hardly fail to come."[69] Reverend Twichell confessed to his father in a letter, "One hardship which our Brigade has encountered is almost too horrible to mention—viz. the stench arising over the dead bodies both of horse and men, lying on the field unburied." He hoped, "The rain will do good, in purifying the air if nothing else."[70] Pvt. James W. Huffman, who joined the Peninsula campaign after serving in the Valley, confirmed that the smell following the battle of Malvern Hill "was almost unendurable" and the "men fell in the ranks."[71] Though soldiers' conception of miasma was inaccurate, the soldiers were wise to link dead bodies to disease.

Both Union and Confederate soldiers also frequently connected contaminated water to poor health. This fear was also savvy, as infected water was the transmitter of diarrhea, the most common illness among soldiers, and also typhoid fever. Water was often contaminated by minerals and deposits or through contact with the byproducts of war, from offal to human waste, and soldiers in camp were forced to imbibe from such putrid sources. Pvt. Oliver Wilcox Norton from Pennsylvania complained that "the climate and exposure, with the bad water, are enough to contend against. Sometimes we have excellent weather, and again we can get nothing but roily swamp water."[72] As in the case of miasma, men tended to detect foul water by its stench. Explained Henry Keiser of the 95th Pennsylvania, "Our drinking water is very poor; it fairly stinks."[73] It took Pvt. Charles Perkins some time to connect his nasty case of diarrhea to the water. At first, he pondered, "Have got Bowel complaint again. Some say it is owing to the water we drink." One month later he confirmed, "Bowels trouble me again owing to water."[74] But other soldiers appeared to catch on more quickly. Sergeant Pryor of Georgia wrote, "I have been quite sick with disintery for four or five days, but am now about well. . . . There is a great deal of [dysentery] in the army here owing, I think, to the water."[75] Pvt. James T. Miller likewise found himself in a "limestone country and the watter is as hard as it can be. and between the hard watter the marching and sleeping in the rain and rob[b]ing us of our rations it made plump [plumb] one half of our regiment sick with the dysentery."[76] While professional physicians quibbled over the causes of diarrhea and dysentery, soldiers observed quite accurately a major source of the problem.

Desperately thirsty men were tempted to drink horrifyingly poor-quality water, despite their suspicions that it would make them sick. Pvt. Kinchen Jahu Carpenter of North Carolina wrote, "It is impossible for me to describe what our troops have gone through. Hunger, thirst and fatigue was awful. We would drink water from a stream that had dead horses in it. When you are so very thirsty, any kind of water is good."[77] W. H. Bird, a private from Alabama en route to Yorktown, recalled in his memoirs, "When the train ran up and halted for us to take the boat, there were a good many that went down to the river to get a drink of water, and when we tasted it was as salty as if you were to fill a cup half full of salt and then fill it with water and stir it up to drink, And all of the vomiting and cursing you ever heard or seen, was down there, for I was in the gang and a participator in the vomiting."[78] Though Bird appeared more amused than disheartened in hindsight, it was much more difficult to maintain one's spirits given the persistently bad water in 1862. As Chaplain Twichell from New York put it, "Heat produces thirst, and the water is so poor, that if drunk freely it produces diarrhea which in turn saps the foundations of spirit and energy."[79] Pvt. Andrew W. Gillett of the 52nd Virginia longed for home, because in his current Valley location, he could not find "any water as good as the worset pond in Bath County."[80] Put simply, poor water inspired homesickness for a bygone time before war had befouled the local supplies.

From insects to rodents, the soldiers lamented pests and the irritations they provoked. The men did not, however, recognize the beasts as alarming transmitters of disease—such as mosquitoes of malaria, lice of typhus, and ticks of Lyme—until the very end of the century when vector-borne disease had been discovered. It is easy to understand, however, why soldiers were so troubled by these constant companions in camp. A louse, for instance, bites in order to feed upon blood, causing an allergic reaction that ignites furious itching. Often sores develop around the armpits, waist, and torso with particular rawness at any point where a clothing seam touches the body. What soldiers did not realize was that itching was the least of their problems: lice transmitted typhus, a disease which causes fever, cough, chills, joint pain, rashes, headaches, delirium, and stupor (often confused with typhoid fever, a different disease spread by fecal contamination).

Growing accustomed to lice was a rite of passage for soldiers, and one that effected swift demoralization and humiliation. As the famous Union memoirist Pvt. John D. Billings termed it, "Like death, [the louse] was no respecter of persons. . . . It inserted its bill as confidingly into the body of the major-general as of the lowest private."[81] Pvt. William A. Fletcher from Texas remembered how he first "drew my hand out from under cover and held it to the light, and there, sure enough, was something alive, for I could see its legs working. . . . Such a feeling of disgrace one rarely has. I made an examination of clothing and bedding and saw that I was well supplied with them of all sizes and nits by the hundreds." He observed, at least in hindsight, that the humiliation lessened as one became seasoned by soldiering. "But as time passed, I got over my feeling of disgrace and learned that we were all subjects, under like conditions."[82] Private Billings agreed that over time embarrassment gave way to "hardened indifference," but "the secretiveness which a man suddenly developed when he found himself inhabited for the first time was very entertaining. He would cuddle all knowledge of it as closely as the old Forty-Niners did the hiding-place of their bag of gold-dust."[83] Private Carter managed to avoid lice for some time, but eventually the close quarters and filth of soldier life got the better of him. "One night I was troubled a good deal by something running about on my neck all night long; I suspected that it was an army of lice, and in the morning I found outside my tent, by my corner (and I sleep close, for there were five in the tent) an old dirty shirt, all covered over with body lice."[84] Irritating and embarrassing, lice were a constant reminder that war changed the environment and the men in it. Lice simply became an omnipresent component of camp filth.

Though soldiers did not consider ticks to be as "unclean" as lice, they too would prove to be disease vectors, and contemporarily, unwelcome companions.[85] Ticks burrow into the skin and can carry several bacterial diseases, leading to fever, aches, and poor appetite, or the more serious Lyme disease, which is characterized by early rash, fatigue, fever, and muscle and joint pain. Modern scholars are not confident Lyme was widespread during the Civil War, but these same scholars have also overlooked the common presence of ticks in the camps.[86] Lieutenant Haydon was quite clear that a major occupation of the Virginia soldier was extracting the pests from their fleshy dens. "We were considerably troubled by gnats & mosquitoes. Woodticks are however our greatest annoyance." Weeks later, he elaborated, "We have to spend an hour every day picking off woodticks." By that point, the soldiers had also acquired other traveling companions: "Most of the men owing to our mode of living & the want of clean clothes are now for the first time becoming lousy." At least soldiers were in good company and helped each other to laugh at their misfortunes: "I heard Prentice say this m'g that he was 'going to make a desperate attempt to drive the enemy from his earth works' meaning that he would try to get the lice & ticks out of his shoes & stockings."[87] Prentice was not the only soldier who described ticks as enemies in war. Rev. A. M. Stewart explained at length, "Under all the dry pine leaves, where we encamp, a great secesh army of wood-ticks have wintered. The late warm weather has waked them into activity, and, after their long fast, hungry as hyenas. Few so happy as not to find each morning half a dozen of these villanous blood-suckers sticking in his flesh." Trying to make light of this misfortune, he continued, "Health prescribers are wont to assert that frequent rubbing and irritation of the skin, is a necessity to good health in a warm climate. Not the slightest fear, therefore, of us in this respect."[88]

Given the swampy state of the Peninsula, it is no wonder that soldiers stationed there complained bitterly about the mosquitoes. Confederate Pvt. James Huffman wrote from White Oak Swamp that "as we marched along through these swamps, the big swamp mosquitoes would stick their long bills through all our clothes, to get a last farewell taste of our blood. Their bills were as long as the tongues of jew's-harps."[89] Rebel Pvt. John Leavitt was alarmed by the blood-suckers he had endured in "white oak swamp when the water was up to my waist." The "mosquitoes [were] as thick as flies in July and August."[90] Interestingly, both of these soldiers were Virginians, and yet they had not encountered such multitudes of mosquitoes in civilian life. The persistent wet weather, the digging for fortifications and camps that left pools of standing water, and the increased time soldiers spent outside without protection likely led to this transformation.

Soldiers resented mosquitoes at the time, but looking back in their memoirs, they fixated upon the insects, particularly after they learned that mosquitoes, not miasma, had been the real carriers of malaria. Reverend Stewart remembered that his "extemporized shanty has been visited by picket-guards and squads of full-grown mosquitoes" despite the earliness of the season.[91] Private Bellard recalled being attacked by an "army of Virginia mosquitoes." He and comrades "were completely surrounded and had to keep our arms continually in motion trying to brush them off."[92] A Confederate chaplain, Rev. Wayland F. Dunaway, wrote his memoir in 1913 after the discovery of mosquito-borne malarial plasmodia by Sir Ronald Ross in 1897. He recast his experience in 1862: "General Johnston posted his army between Richmond and the Chickahominy river . . . in the pestilential low-grounds of that sluggish stream. Swarms of mosquitoes attacked us at night and with their hypodermic proboscides injected poisonous malaria in our veins, to avoid which the sleeping soldier covered his head with a blanket." He described how the "complexion of the men became sallow, and every day numbers of the men were put on the sick-list by the surgeons."[93]

Last but not least among insects were the dreaded swarms of flies that gravitated to the death, wounds, and disease that clung to the armies. Flies were also unseen spreaders of bacteria that would stick to their feet and bodies and transmit typhoid, dysentery, and diarrhea to human flesh, food, and water. Private Leavitt complained about "how [the flies] do bite me while I am writing this [letter]," while Pvt. Allen Seymour Davis of Minnesota, stationed at Harrison's Landing in August, grumbled that flies were the "greatest annoyance we have." They flew into his mouth each time he opened it for a bite of food.[94] After the Seven Days battles, Private Fletcher aptly remembered how fighting could precipitate a rush of flies. As the men were "passing over and near the battlefield, seeing the destruction that it brought to man, beast and property," they suffered from "the awful stench that at times would great one's nostrils, and in this instance myriads of flies." In Fletcher's remembrance, these were not your everyday flies. "They were something less than the common housefly, and when they bit or sucked it left a stinging sensation, and when one lay down for a nap in daytime he was forced to cover up, as it were, head and ears."[95] Reverend Stewart, who described all manner of insects in illuminating detail in his memoir, also devoted a number of paragraphs in homage to flies. "Whatever comparisons might be instituted between the Egyptians and the Secesh, one thing is certain, the banks of the James river produce flies, as well as those of the Nile." Again employing the language of enemy, "Here we have flies in regiments, in brigades, in divisions, and in corps, great armies of flies—big flies and little flies, biting flies and sucking flies—wood, field and tent flies—night flies and day flies—rising up or lying down, going out or coming in,—in all places and conditions— FLIES." Like Seymour he complained that "whatever kind of food you get prepared to eat, a hungry legion of flies is ever ready to lend a helping hand."[96] Given the regularity with which flies traversed from latrines to food, it was truly a feat to avoid contracting disease.

Sundry other animal pests shared the men's food and disturbed their sleep as well. Pvt. George Perkins from New York recorded, "Slept in a barn with some of the 5th Michigan regt. Barn full of rats. Slept very poorly." He connected the incident with a mysterious rash a few days later: "Found I had caught a kind of itch the night I laid in the corn barn."[97] More likely, Perkins's rash was the common solider itch now believed to have been scabies, a contagious skin disease introduced by tiny mites that burrow into the flesh and deposit their eggs in human hosts. Still, soldiers felt dread at being the close companions of animals they had typically avoided in civilian life. Rats were indeed harbingers of disease, transmitting bacterial and parasitic disease. Pests of amphibious and reptilious makeup also slithered and hopped among the camps. In a more amusing anecdote, Capt. Eugene Blackford of Alabama wrote, "I slept in a swamp where the frogs made night hideous—I have never seen so many in all my life before. They were seen in the trees. I placed 3 fence rails against a fence for a bed,

& this escaped the water which was every where, but the frogs were hopping over my blanket all night, & would sit on me to sing."[98] In the midst of this cacophony, Blackford missed a night of sleep. In May, Pvt. Thomas Landers of the 16th Massachusetts explained to his parents that Suffolk was overrun with snakes: "we arrived here Sunday morning at ten o clock after a march of twenty seven miles. This is the meanest damned hole I have seen & it is hotter than hell here and any quantity of snakes of every description."[99] Soldiers would simply have to learn to live with the snakes. Army operations and combat disrupted many animals from their habitats and put them in contact with the soldiers. The frogs and snakes may not have made soldiers sick, but they did test soldiers' mental resolve. In moments of weakness, men like Landers grew agonizingly homesick.

Taken together, the soldiers' accounts connected environmental factors to sickness and morale. Rebels and Federals stationed in two very different regions identified the same sources of their health problems with little variation. Further, Virginians seemed equally stunned by nature's onslaughts, despite their familiarity with the area. Over time, experience caused some men to call into question their former beliefs about disease environments, while other experiences confirmed presumptions. It is also important to note that while soldiers most often fixated upon the negative impacts of environment on health, they did occasionally suggest its positive effects. On June 16, 1862, 45th Georgia infantryman Pvt. Marion H. Fitzpatrick wrote, "There is much sickness in our Regiment, but we have beautiful weather now and I hope the general health will improve rapidly now."[100] Thus good weather could promote well-being. It could also improve morale; as Private Blackington reported in a letter home to Massachusetts from near Yorktown, "We have very pleasant weather out here now. It seems like summer. We have the merry birds singing their sweet melodious songs in the beautiful trees."[101] Soldiers relaxed and forgot their miseries under fine conditions.

While it was more common for soldiers to praise the beauty of the Valley, allowing the bucolic scenery to boost their spirits, soldiers on the Peninsula also sought out tranquil landscapes to raise morale. Union Surgeon Thomas Ellis wrote, "The region of the James is high, hilly, and bountifully marked by nature with all that vegetable opulence can supply. The ripe wheat-fields, and the long wavy stretches of clover, burst like a vision in fever upon the weary eyes of our wounded and footsore." The soldiers reacted with thanksgiving. "Some fell down by the banks of the river, and lapped the bright water like dogs. Others fell upon the margin, and wept."[102] This description may be over-indulgent, but it does convey the relief soldiers experienced at the sight of an idyllic setting endowed with fresh water.

PHYSICAL AND MENTAL HEALTH IN SUMMARY

One of the benefits of analyzing individual soldier accounts from the winter of 1861–1862 through mid-August 1862 is that it is possible to note each self-reported instance of illness and change in spirits. Doing so confirms what historians have long suspected—that Union official records and the scattered Confederate records vastly underestimated the numbers of sick soldiers in the ranks. For reasons examined in the next chapter, many soldiers either failed to report at morning sick call or were turned away without being recorded as ill, skewing official statistics. The military had no accurate way to gauge mental health, so the contours of soldier attitudes is lost to the historical record unless recovered from eyewitness accounts. A brief comparison of official records (namely the Union records, because they are more complete) to the soldiers' sample in this study reveals that the Virginia-based armies were crippled by widespread, persistent sickness and that army morale was highly capricious. We as scholars have a long way to go to accumulate reliable measurements of Civil War mental and physical health.[103]

The Union records kept track of many illnesses that the soldiers considered environmental or partially environmental in origin and are therefore relevant to this study. These official categories included miasmatic diseases (the fevers), dietetic diseases (such as scurvy), constitutional diseases (such as rheumatism), tubercular and other lung diseases, parasitic diseases (such as worms), so-called local diseases (anything from insanity to headache), and diseases of the digestive organs. The U.S. Medical Department estimated in the Valley from January to June 1862 a total of 18,277 cases of miasmatic diseases, 3,676 cases of digestive organ diseases, 1,979 cases of rheumatism, 344 cases of headache, 6 cases of sunstroke, 34 cases of worms, and 47 cases of scurvy.[104] It is striking that fevers ranked above diarrhea when there is clear evidence that diarrhea was the most common sickness of Civil War soldiers.[105] With a mortality rate of around ten percent, bowel complaints would prove the number-one killer by war's end.[106] Diarrhea was probably underreported because it was so common that surgeons did not bother to count every case, and sick men did not report it unless incapacitated. On the Peninsula, there was a similar distortion. During the same period, there were 135,433 cases of miasma, 36,113 of diarrhea, 18,526 of rheumatism, 2753 of headache,

125 of sunstroke, 515 of worms, and 1,114 of scurvy.[107] These numbers appear higher than those from the Valley in part because of the larger army present on the Peninsula, but also because there were proportionately slightly more cases of sickness on the Peninsula. Different seasons did inspire spikes in different types of illness; for instance, respiratory ailments such as catarrh (inflammation of the mucous membranes) and pneumonia were more prevalent in the cold months and diarrhea and malaria in the warm months.[108] In the Confederacy, regimental records include an equally vast number of possible environmental ailments: fevers, bowel complaints, respiratory diseases, brain and nervous system disorders, venereal diseases, and disorders of virtually all body parts. Unlike the Union, the still underreported diarrhea and dysentery were found to be most prevalent, though often closely followed by miasmatic diseases in the 1862 monthly reports.[109] Again, Confederate records exist only at the regimental level and give little overall sense of numbers given that health varied widely from regiment to regiment.[110]

The portrait of physical health in the Confederate and Union armies in this sample was almost identical. Diarrhea was the most common ailment described for both sides, followed by fevers, then rheumatic aches and pains. Forty-three percent of soldiers from both sides described themselves or their regiments as being in extremely poor health during the campaigns from January to mid-August 1862, meaning they suffered frequent debilitating illnesses or prolonged periods of inefficacy or hospitalization. These soldiers were too sick to be reliable in the ranks, often straggling to rest or seek care, repeatedly reporting to sick call or the hospital, and unable to fulfill their daily duties. Eleven percent of soldiers described their health as fair, suffering several incidents of acute sickness that took them out of duty for days, but they were able to return to effective duty. This is compared to the fifteen percent who described good health, with only the occasional and minor headache, cold, or intestinal distress, or who reported no evidence of illness during the eight months of the sample. As mentioned, in the early spring men were sicker in the Valley, and for the rest of the period men were sicker on the Peninsula.[111]

Soldiers who self-reported tended to identify weather as the primary contributor to poor health. Exposure coupled with exhaustion was probably a greater underlying cause of illness in the Valley than on the Peninsula. This explains the early spike in disease in the Valley in March, when weather was at its most mercurial. On the Peninsula, exposure was also extreme but movement less so; therefore, miasma appeared more threatening to the men, though insects were the hidden culprits behind malaria. Stagnancy also contributed to typhoid fever, transmitted through the soiled waters of immobile army camps. Disease was thus worse on the Peninsula in the hot, humid later spring and summer months—June through August—when insects were at their thickest and water quality at its worst.[112]

While it may seem to make sense that Southerners, or more rightly Virginians, would have already been better adjusted and bodily acclimated to the environmental challenges of the commonwealth, the evidence suggests that being a Virginian yielded little to no physical or mental advantage. Environmental experience in wartime was not as simple as in peace, when being accustomed to the muggy heat of summer or having already contracted and survived falciparum malaria might have been a major advantage. The reality of camp life was that having immunity to one type of malaria would in no way preclude catching other dangerous fevers, such as typhoid. If a Virginian could heartily withstand a ninety-degree day in sweltering humidity on the farm, in war he was forced to do this without bathing or washing his clothes, sleeping on the ground, or perhaps enduring a grueling twenty-mile march. There was no comparison. The advantage the Southerner from Georgia might have possessed in weathering summer was his disadvantage in the winter, while Northerners and Midwesterners found the Virginia winters to be balmy compared to what they had experienced at home. Thus, previous experiences were variable and only sporadically amounted to fleeting advantages.

Unlike physical health, mental health was not carefully documented in official records, because it was difficult for nineteenth-century surgeons to categorize. Lacking an extensive vocabulary for mental disorders, physicians used the diagnosis of nostalgia to encompass a number of mental maladies, or if mental distress was especially marked, mania (a Confederate category) or insanity. But even as a catchall, nostalgia was of real concern to military operations, because it appeared accompanied by physical symptoms and in some cases proved fatal. According to the *Medical and Surgical History of the War of the Rebellion*, from January to June in the Shenandoah Valley U.S. soldiers suffered 118 reported cases of nostalgia. It is important to note that these cases were severe to the point of complete debilitation and removal from the frontlines; those suffering from lesser cases of homesickness or melancholy would not have been reported. In addition, nine cases of insanity and at least one suicide appeared in the records. For the Army of the Potomac on the Peninsula during this same period, 133 were reported as suffering from nostalgia, 174 from insanity, and twelve ended their lives voluntarily.[113] The numbers so vastly underrepresented self-reported low morale that official records might be useful only to suggest that the U.S. Medical Department acknowledged that mental afflictions existed. The numbers on the Confederate side are extremely difficult to amass, but a sample of Confederate regimental medical records reveal that a comparable few soldiers suffered from "nostalgia" and "mania," the only two mental categories Rebel surgeons recorded.[114]

The sample taken for this study is more reflective of the range of minor to serious mental afflictions soldiers suffered in 1862 than the official records. Approximately twenty-two percent of the men expressed frequent homesickness, loneliness, melancholy, and despair in 1862, resulting in significant impairment to army operations. An additional five percent (often officers) worried constantly about morale in the ranks, even if they maintained their own spirits, and an additional twelve percent suffered from at least occasional attacks of the blues. This is significant considering that around forty percent of the men surveyed did not explicitly mention spirits.[115]

Every human suffers from occasional sadness; thus, when attempting to understand exactly how melancholy translated into lowered morale and reduced army efficiency, it can be useful to look beyond words to actions. As Pvt. Gerald Fitzgerald of the 12th Massachusetts put it to his sweetheart, "I hardly know why I take my pen uninspired to write to you unless to provoke an answer for, as I suppose I must have often told you, letters are all I have. . . . For news of me take blank and divide by ten and you have my shadow that I am forced to call my life." He could scarcely remove himself from his tent to attend to duties. "We of the Army of nothing and nobody, Head Quarters no-where, on duty against the Commissary Department, may afterall, settle the 'on to Richmond' clamor by obeying the 'Vox Populi,'" he continued, apparently losing interest in the cause.[116] The morale of Alfred L. Castleman, a surgeon in the 5th Wisconsin, appeared to be sinking as he wrote, "The hardships which we suffer in this world, instead of awakening a sympathy for others in the same condition, are more apt to call up unworthy comparisons, with a remark, that 'they need not complain; they are no worse off than we are.'" So worn down was Castleman by camp conditions that he could scarcely think of anything positive to say when writing home. "Try . . . long camping and disappointed expectations, amid the swamps of the Chickahominy, living on half rations of hard crackers and salt beef, and you will then be able to appreciate the hardships of dry food, and the difficulty of assimulating from it moist ideas."[117] Though he jested, Castleman's sunken spirits, made worse by the tremendous burden of responsibility for soldier health, prompted the surgeon to defy army discipline in several trivial matters, result[ing in] his court martial.[118] In this manner could low morale lead to diminish[ed] resolve to follow orders and dissatisfaction with military structures.

Alcoholism was another sign that low spirits made for unreliable soldiers. Doctors often prescribed whiskey as treatment for ills, but there were soldiers who used liquor beyond its medicinal benefits. In White Oak Swamp, Pvt. Fred Laubach of Pennsylvania went on an early morning binge after a particularly rough night: "This morning we were aroused pretty early. Being wet and cold we could not sleep so we built a fire and warmed up, got our whiskey, eat our breakfast. . . . I had three rations of whiskey which made me a little tipsy. Bull for that."[119] Though perhaps warm at last, Laubach was not fit for duty by the end of breakfast. The unpleasant duty of rooting out the drunkards in the ranks fell to the officers. As Virginia artillerist Capt. Edward Rush Young explained, "Off Day rainy & sleety anticipated a dismal night for visiting the various pickets. Had the disagreeable duty of examining the cabins for liquor with orders to pour it out wherever found as some peaceable men complained of being disturbed by a drunken frolic the night before. Found none however as they are always smart enough to hide it."[120] Not just the rabble turned to drink for comfort in the midst of environmental torment. A Catholic chaplain guiltily confessed his reliance on alcohol to his fellows back home, as he accompanied the Confederate army on the Peninsula: "But do you know what I do to preserve my precious health? I'll tell you in a low voice. Now don't be scandalized, and whatever you do, don't tell anyone else. I've been taking w-h-i-s-k-e-y." He then attempted to diminish the scandal, "Of course, I don't like it and I never will. But certain trustworthy people assure me that it is a *sine-qua-non* for the life I lead. Hence reason dictates, despite the taste, that I finish off a bottle every ten days. At any rate, it will never make me fat!"[121] Subsequent letters revealed that his colleagues were not impressed with his behavior.

The ultimate act of mental debility was suicide.[122] The men who took their own lives were probably suffering from severe mental health problems, some that preceded the war. Contemporaries, however, sometimes believed that suicide occurred when a man could not adapt to the realities of soldiering. One 18th Massachusetts soldier remembered that in January 1862, "Private Booth of Company A, entered the guard tent, hung the trigger of his musket over a nail, put the muzzle to his breast and sent three buckshot and a bullet through his body. We knew that he was despondent: that he said he had rather be dead than to be a soldier, but never dreamed of his ending his enlistment in this manner."[123] A hospital worker described the heartbreaking illness of hundreds of men

f Williamsburg, followed by several attempted and two

s as men hurled themselves into the water to end their

ey campaign a well-known suicide occurred in April

Holliday shot himself in the head. As David Hunter

..., a federal soldier from Virginia, wrote, "Was informed that Colonel Holliday of the Vermont cavalry had committed suicide, the cause said to be disgust with the bad discipline of his regiment." More likely the cause of Holliday's suicide lay within Strother's description of the man's demeanor, suggesting extreme distress. Holliday was "a tall man with a huge beard and of a melancholy mien, talking rarely and in monosyllables. I was introduced to him three days ago and remarked on his sad and speechless demeanor. He ordered his regiment to march and remaining behind lit his pipe and blew his brains out."[125] General Banks confirmed the incident in his official report on April 6, 1862. "The death of Colonel Holliday was very sudden and very sad. He appeared greatly depressed when here about the condition of his regiment, which was then at Strasburg." Further, "his officers say he had been nearly insane for three weeks, and attribute his depression of spirits to personal disappointments not connected with his profession. I do not know why this may be. His death occurred near Strasburg, while he was near the head of his column. He shot himself in the head, and died without a word."[126] It would be silly to suggest that environmental adversity alone contributed to suicide, but the daily discomfort of soldiering and prolonged separation from loved ones in combination with combat trauma tested the limits of those in poor mental condition.

To sum up this soldier experience in the 1862 Peninsula and Shenandoah Valley campaigns, soldiers perceived nature as tremendously hampering to mental and physical health. They based their assessments on what they observed and experienced, coming to useful if sometimes fragmented conclusions about the sources of their distress. Their environmental suffering was influenced not only by the changes wartime brought to the landscape but by the larger realities of army life. Exposure to environmental illness was compounded by supply problems, army regulations, camping, marching, and other aspects of soldiering that were not under the men's control but rather managed by commanders, officers, and medical personnel. It was to this official network of care that soldiers were supposed to turn to prevent and treat their illness and melancholy. But the army health care system would prove deeply dissatisfying.

3

Soldiers and Official Military
Health Care

Before the war, common soldiers could scarcely have imagined the sprawling, alien medical systems that would be constructed by the United States
and the Confederacy. Properly supporting soldier health necessitated the
consideration of supply lines and camp sanitation, sick call and diagnostic
procedures in the ranks, treatment at regimental and remote hospitals,
and rehabilitation. Because of the division of labor in military bureaucracy,
not all these elements were under the purview of the two sides' Medical
Departments. The health systems of the Union and Confederacy involved
the Quartermaster and Commissary Departments, commanding generals, military and medical officers, the presidents, and, in the case of the
United States, the civilians of the U.S. Sanitary Commission — composed of
elite social and medical reformers, middle-class male and female reformers, and average Northerners at home. Meanwhile, Union and Confederate civilians scrutinized medical progress and commented upon it in the
newspapers, pushing for changes that might preserve the health of their
loved ones. It is no surprise, then, that this complex network of individuals quarreled over power, conflicting medical theories, and varying obli-
gations. Further, even the brightest, most forward-thinking health care
workers only dimly comprehended environmental management, disease
prevention, and medical treatment. Even so, institutional obstacles were
more crippling to health care in 1862 than were individuals. These factors
involved a shortage of staff, supplies, and hospitals and the painfully gradual nature of reform endemic to democracies. Despite the complex tangle
of problems, both Medical Departments were able to institute reform
programs that would improve soldier health over time, if not drastically

during the 1862 Peninsula and Shenandoah Valley campaigns; however, in the first year and a half of war, taking responsibility for one's own body was not only an accepted cultural convention, it was vital to survival.

Increased contact with the unfamiliar did not lead soldiers to heightened confidence in science or trust in the Medical Departments in 1862; quite the contrary.[1] Common soldiers often criticized and sometimes rejected a system of care they found ineffectual, impersonal, and even condemnatory given the class differences with some of their caretakers. They leveled their harshest critiques at surgeons, assistant surgeons, hospital stewards, nurses, and military officers.[2] In return, common soldiers were often viewed as low-class, undisciplined volunteers in need of guidance by the enlightened middle and upper classes. To a certain extent, the opinion was justifiable. Officers were supposed to regulate and train their troops not only to prepare them for combat, but also to preserve their health. And yet middle-class paternalism spread beyond securing army efficiency to enforcing a code of expected behavior, evident particularly in the newspapers. This feedback loop increased estrangement between soldiers and civilians.

SOLDIERS ASSESS THE OFFICIAL NETWORK OF CARE

"Against entering an hospital, there usually exists in the mind of the soldier a strong repugnance, even a manifest horror. Nor is this, by any means, an unnatural feeling," wrote Union chaplain A. M. Stewart.[3] Though Stewart believed he was speaking on behalf of the common soldier, and in some sense he was, his comments better reflected his middle-class origins. According to Stewart's parameters for proper behavior, soldiers should fear hospitals, because "too often they are cold, heartless places, to which, even when sick, the soldier is carried with great reluctance. As a consequence, the good soldier is wont to resist and stave off an approaching disease as long as possible, by a performance of ordinary duties." As historian Frances Clarke's *War Stories* has elucidated, forbearing in one's pain earned a man cultural clout in a society coping with mass suffering.[4] Indeed, as Stewart wrote, "When finally forced to yield, the bravest and strongest usually gives up altogether,—lie down in the cheerless, homeless tent, draw up their blanket over their head, and almost refuse to move, until forced away by command of an officer."[5] Here Stewart elaborated that the respectable soldier, in an embrace of striking individualism, would refuse altogether to succumb to army medical infrastructures unless compelled by direct order. The fact that Stewart had class-specific expectations for the men's behavior does not mean he lacked genuine compassion. It fell to chaplains to spiritually comfort soldiers, and in doing so many grew terribly impressed by the hardships soldiers suffered. But chaplains and aid workers often did have different priorities than common soldiers, some of which went beyond keeping the men healthy.[6]

While middle-class Americans cast the conflict between enlisted men and their medical systems in moral terms, common soldiers appeared less concerned about how well they performed at suffering and were instead reluctant to engage with the Medical Departments because they feared the unknown. Because so few Americans had been treated in a hospital before the war, accustoming oneself to hospital care required a distinct shift in cultural values. Soldiers missed home care and their loved ones, particularly women, to whom they had always turned in the past. Stewart did observe this fact when he attempted to cheer up a sick soldier, who did not wish to go to a hospital. "Though neither home nor friends had been mentioned, I said abruptly: 'My dear friend, you are homesick.' 'O,' he exclaimed, as the big tears filled his eyes, 'home is every thought.'"[7] Common soldiers were explicit about their trepidation over this cultural shift. Pvt. Albert M. Liscom of the 13th Massachusetts explained, "I pity the man who is sick in the army. The army is nothing but a mill to grind the life and soul out of a man."[8] Pvt. Kinchen Jahu Carpenter of the 50th North Carolina adamantly preferred home care to the hospital in Petersburg, and even regimental surgeons admitted missing the healing touch of loved ones.[9] As Union surgeon Alfred L. Castleman wrote, "How much I miss the tender care of my family in sickness." Even when he recovered from illness, he continued to feel "sad."[10] In lieu of family, soldiers feared separation from their units, as volunteer regiments were raised locally and composed of familiar faces, their closest links to home.

Before visiting a hospital for the first time, green soldiers succumbed to rumors of mistreatment, echoed by the apprehensions of loved ones at home. Eliza Howard, for instance, imagined a scenario of fantastical neglect in a letter to her husband. "We hear every now and then of some new abuse among the surgeons, regular and volunteer, —for instance: Mr. Hopkins told us of one poor fellow of a Vermont regiment who was brought to the hospital in Alexandria with typhoid fever, having both feet frozen and one of them eaten by rats! It is too horrible to think of."[11] The story conveys not only her mistrust of a system of which she was ignorant but her helplessness at being deprived of the role women had once almost exclusively performed in their loved ones' lives. The displacement of care from private to public venue meant that hospital professionals would have less of a vested interest in comforting the individual than family members, who were most concerned with a soldier's health and happiness. This reality greatly contributed to the appeal of the U.S. Sanitary Commission, which enabled civilian access to soldier health care in both direct and indirect ways and contributed to the Commission's war-long evolution toward increased focus on the individual soldier.[12] Meanwhile, it is important to bear in mind that regimental surgeons were often raised locally with their men and therefore were more likely to be an acquaintance, further contributing to soldiers' desires to be treated within the ranks rather than removed to a hospital.

As far as soldiers were concerned, once in a hospital they often had their worst fears confirmed. Musician Lewis Shepard succumbed to that fate and lay in bed for over two weeks, "not getting any better." Like many in his circumstances, "I have been in hopes that the Authorities would discharge me or send me home till I got fit for service again. One thing is certain I cannot get well here."[13] Their spirits plunged, compounded by the fact of being suddenly surrounded by hundreds of the sick and wounded. Pvt. W. H. Bird was party to a small pox outbreak at a Danville, Virginia, hospital. The senior surgeon ordered, "Close the doors and not let a one go to the army that we have here. Better to let this 80 die than to send them back to camps and the disease they carry with them, kill, maybe 10,000 others." From the doctor's perspective quarantining the hospital would save precious lives to carry on the war effort, but to Bird the implication was chillingly callous.[14] His life, so precious to his family members, had become expendable.

The soldiers were also more carefully scrutinized by hospital workers than they would have been by family members. The middle to upper classes believed in their own superior capacities to deal with suffering and death, and they pushed soldiers to conform to their conceptions.[15] Even Castleman, who at one point was a regimental surgeon and quite sympathetic toward common soldiers, wrote, "I have witnessed cases of 'hospital gangrene,' low typhoid fevers, with gangrenous toes or fingers dropping off. . . . 'Twas a gangrene of the mind, for want of free ventilation of the brain. There is no disease so contagious, or so depressing to vital energy when taken, as inactivity and gloominess of mind." Castleman thus made it his goal to pass through his hospital eliciting "a hearty laugh" from each patient. "I think my hospital can boast, just now, the happiest set of sick men I ever saw," he declared, noting the effects of recreation and games on positive thinking. "This morning, as I was prescribing for them, (all sitting up) some reading the morning papers, and talking loudly over war news, some playing whist, some checkers, some chess, some dominoes—all laughing and merry." He concluded, "They are all the better for these things, and when I return them to their quarters, they take hold of their work with a will."[16] By this typical middle-class chain of thought, men who persevered in suffering would go on to be more efficient contributors to the war effort. Nurse Sarah Edmonds similarly observed, "I noticed that whenever I failed to arouse a man from such a state of feeling [bad for himself], it generally proved a hopeless case. They were very likely to die, and persisted in believing that there was no alternative."[17] A soldier therefore had a personal responsibility to improve his odds of survival; if he died, his negative attitude was partly to blame. This conception of soldier suffering also permeated the ranks of the U.S. Sanitary Commission. Commission nurse Katherine Wormeley encouraged a fever-ridden Pennsylvanian: "'What a terribly long face,' said I, trying to rally him; 'you will never get well till you learn to laugh.'"[18] Common soldiers were steeped in these values as they flooded the hospitals and some came to parrot the sentiments. For instance, a Confederate soldier from Alabama explained, "I soon learned . . . that a strong resolution was equal to a good constitution. . . . Nine cases out of ten whenever a sick soldier yielded to the idea that he would not recover, he certainly would die."[19] But this did not change the fact that the heightened scrutiny of the hospital environment wore on the men and informed their preference for care outside the official military network.

While soldiers often favored their regimental surgeons, whom they may or may not have known from home, many still questioned their surgeons' motivations and abilities and the efficacy of their prescriptions. Some enlisted men felt they were unceremoniously denied care at morning sick call, such as Pvt. G. Q. French. "D—m that Dr. I'll hunt him till he caves. As if I don't know when I am sick," he wrote after being returned to duty quite ill. The next day he made the doctor believe he was sick and did receive medication.[20] Further, soldiers' encounters with surgeons and their arsenal of chemical medications did little to convince the men that science was superior to practical knowledge. Many soldiers experienced the medications they received as inadequate. Sgt. Henry Keiser of Pennsylvania, who suffered from diarrhea for a month, finally visited his surgeon, leading only to disappointment. "I got two pills and a dose of vil from the Doctor which made me very sick all day."[21] Pvt. Irvin Fox of Indiana, stricken with a swelling head and neck, complained, "Doctor calls it Neuralgia but can do nothing for me at present." A diagnosis was of no use to Fox without a remedy. This is not to say that Fox was particularly fond of medication. Indeed, his earlier case of violent diarrhea had been treated with "four monstrous large quinine powders whitch is rather poor medicine for soldiers who have to sleep on the damp ground & are exposed to nearly every rain storm."[22] In short, Fox felt the doctor failed to get to the bottom of what ailed him: environmental exposure. He was not interested in the surgeon's science; he was interested in relief.

In many cases, the prescribed heroic interventions appeared worse than soldiers' initial diseases. Lieutenant Haydon, for instance, did not thank his surgeon for the medicine he received at sick call that "stopped the diarhoae" but resulted in him vomiting "no less than eleven times to day."[23] Pvt. Aaron E. Bachman blamed his surgeon for causing his "swamp fever" to become critical. The doctor "gave me ten or fifteen grains of quinine and a lump of bluemass [a preparation of mercury and often licorice, herbs, and sugar] as big as a cherry, and required me to take it in his presence." In consequence, "the intense heat, the fever, and the doctor's 'dope' fixed me completely, so I gave my blacksmith's tools away and was taken to the hospital," and his worst fear turned into reality. By the time Bachman reached the hospital, he was almost dead from exposure.[24] Pvt. Oscar Bailey of the 1st Massachusetts wrote bitterly that "all the falt is now in the doctors for when we get sick they do not know how to take care of us they have no medicine nor they do not intend to take care of us."[25]

This is not to say that soldiers never appreciated their surgeons or that it was only their humble roots that made them doubt the science underlying professional treatment. Some welcomed their surgeons as friends from home, and many were grateful for a "kind" doctor.[26] Soldiers indeed recognized that not all surgeons were created equal. The replacement of an inept surgeon was greeted with relief by the entire regiment: "I herd this week that our old Sergeon Dr. Green was dismissed & there will be another in his place soon: I think it a good thing for the regiment."[27] And it is worth noting that the middle class also experienced frustration with the lack of understanding surgeons possessed about disease. One chaplain wrote, "After a week of fatigue, general malaise and a touch of dysentery, I decided to go to the hospital on the day before Pentecost. . . . I'm as weak as a cat, and I've been having headaches which the doctors cannot explain any more than I can."[28]

While soldiers were predisposed to be suspicious of the intentions of military medical staff, Union soldiers were more accepting of the civilian component of their official care network, namely in the form of the U.S. Sanitary Commission. Operating in conjunction with the U.S. Medical Bureau and using military logistical networks, the Sanitary Commission would reach Union soldiers in several direct ways in 1862 Virginia: by providing additional medical staff and hospitals, by distributing goods directly to the men, and by inspecting camps to provide reports on how to improve soldier health. While Commission nurses and doctors tended to blend in with other workers in the hospitals, the members who roamed army camps reminded soldiers of the care of loved ones. For instance, prominent Commission member Fredcrick N. Knapp described in his diary a typical day in the field, distributing goods on June 14, 1862, near Richmond. First thing in the morning, he made arrangements for the sick and wounded to receive supplies as they boarded trains for hospitals near White House Landing. Next, he distributed whiskey, blankets, hospital shirts, oranges, quinine, sherry, guava jelly, lemons, tea, fly nets, and farina to several regiments and their hospitals.[29] These goods were either things soldiers missed from home or added considerably to their protection and comfort. In such ways were Commission workers among the soldiers, supporting the individual health of the men much like home care would have done. Commission inspectors also tangibly improved soldiers' daily lives by making concrete recommendations to the War Department that mitigated environmental exposure and encouraged sanitation. For instance, Pvt. Ephraim Wood, a Union soldier in the Valley, noted that "the Sanitary Committee were here day before yesterday. They condemned these ponchos tents and we have been ordered to make out requisitions for Libby tents, which will add to our comfort a good deal."[30] A soldier from the 16th Massachusetts summed up his feelings of gratitude for the Commission: "This noble agency for the relief of sick, wounded, or destitute soldiers, continues earnestly and faithfully its kind and judicious labors. . . . I have never praised it before, for lack of this previous examination." But now, "I desire now to add my hearty and sincere testimony as to the wisdom, energy, and kindness of the action of the Sanitary Commission. After viewing its operations, I hardly see how the army could have existed without it." In a final surge of enthusiasm, he finished, "God bless all who care for the soldier away from his home and its comforts."[31]

Non-combatants and civilians at home also praised the Commission's efforts in the ranks, recognizing the Commission's special efforts to aid the individual. Chaplain Twichell, for instance, wrote his father, "The Sanitary Commission has done a great deal to mitigate the evil where they could get at it, yet there can hardly be said to be any cooperation in the matter, for the feeling displayed by Army Medical Officers toward this institution is anything but cordial." He did worry, however, that because of internal conflict, "the Commission has been somewhat deflected from its original design and does not have an eye single to human considerations."[32] Twichell was thus enthusiastic about the Commission's early efforts but feared the army's influence. Many of the civilians at home had personal connections to the Commission, as they donated goods or gradually began to use the Commission's services to locate their loved ones in hospitals or cemeteries. Among "acknowledgements" collected in the Commission's final report on Washington Hospital in 1866, an anonymous civilian praised, "I have received three letters from you which is certainly taking a great deal of trouble in behalf of a perfect stranger and I must express my sincere gratitude for your disinterested kindness." Another wrote, "Your kindness and friendship . . . has won our lasting gratitude, and we will say as thousands throughout the land, in saying 'God Bless the Sanitary Commission.'"[33] The Commission had an active interest in eliciting sympathy from soldiers and the public via newspaper articles and its own newsletter, the *Sanitary Bulletin*, which began publication in 1863. Just as the Commission relied solely upon civilian donations, it also required their confidence that the Sanitary Commission was a worthwhile undertaking.[34] It also afforded its members power and prestige within the war effort, which speaks to Twichell's suspicion that Commission workers' intentions may not have been entirely altruistic.

Soldiers recognized that military and civilian medical staff were not the only people involved in the official network of care. Their military officers could have a major influence over their health, for better or for worse. According to army regulations, various officers had responsibilities for locating, laying out, and overseeing the sanitation of camp (including managing garbage and latrines) and for supervising dress and personal hygiene. While the instructions generally included health as a consideration (sometimes too generally to be very instructive), they also explicitly subordinated health mandates to military imperatives. For instance, the camping party of a regiment (consisting of the regimental quartermaster, quartermaster-sergeant, a corporal, and two men) were responsible for scouting a camp location with adequate water. The regulations called for the camping party to examine the "watering-places" and place "signals at those deemed dangerous."[35] The explanation was both under-detailed about what constituted adequate, not to mention clean, water and also, quite sensibly, ranked protection as top priority. Hence, even the proper execution of this task might have led to a lack of water or impure sources, let alone if officers were inept. Another example of inadequate army regulations had to do with camp design. Regulations stipulated that sinks (latrines) were to be 150 paces in front of the color line (or to the rear or flank) for enlisted men and 100 paces to the rear of camp for the officers. In addition to being close to camps, latrines were dangerously near to the kitchens, which resided twenty paces to the rear of the tents. Rainstorms could easily lead to contamination even at the most carefully laid out camps. A common latrine trench was approximately ten to twelve feet long, one to two feet wide, and six to eight feet deep—an area quickly filled by the hundreds of men assigned to its use. In order to preserve the sanitation of the latrines, the regulations fixed that "a portion of the earth dug out for sinks [was] to be thrown back occasionally," and when the bulk of the sink was filled to one and a half to two feet from the top, it was retired.[36] It was difficult, given the pace of a campaign or terrain of a region, for officers to always follow the regulations to the letter even if they were familiar with them. Because most Civil War officers were volunteers, it took some time for them to learn their official duties.

While soldiers did not always understand the nuances of army regulations, they tended to praise officers who were attentive to sanitation.[37] Cpl. Washington Hands of the Confederate 1st Maryland was thankful for the careful instruction of an conscientious officer. He commended his "commander in his efforts to promote the health & comfort of those placed under his charge," believing that "the most rigid Sanitary regulations [were] adapted for the camp; and . . . the neat appearance and healthy condition of the men contrasted with that of other regiments around us."[38] Pvt. William C. McClellan noted, "Our company has had as little sickness as most companys because Capt. H[obbs] makes the men keep clean."[39]

The occasional soldier did balk at the rigidity of sanitary protocol in the army. As volunteers, some soldiers found themselves reluctant to engage in some of the more public displays of hygiene required in such close quarters, such as using the latrines or group bathing. Unless compelled by officers, certain men, especially new recruits, preferred privacy and straggled to obtain it. In turn, some officers disciplined the derelict. For instance, as punishment for forgoing the latrines, an officer might force an offender to wear a barrel shirt upon which feces were stacked just inches from his nose.[40] Thus, not all attempts of officers to protect health were warmly received.

ORIGINS AND EVOLUTION OF THE 1862 MEDICAL INFRASTRUCTURES

As the soldiers were only dimly aware, 1862 was a critical year in the development of Union and Confederate infrastructures to accommodate the ballooning numbers of sick and wounded. The year brought a number of improvements to both Medical Departments in terms of organization, logistics, hospitals, and staff, contributing to a health care system that was measurably superior to that which had served soldiers in the Mexican-American War.[41] Many of the developments, however, had to do with attending to the wounded rather than the sick, and only some of the changes addressed the environmental problems that soldiers viewed as contributing to poor health. Further, constructing army health care was a contentious project, especially in the United States, which had the larger and more established bureaucracy and the additional civilian arm of the U.S. Sanitary Commission.

In 1861, the Union appeared to possess the advantage in assembling a robust army Medical Department. With a larger population to draw upon and more chemical manufactures and supplies, it did retain the necessary resources. Its Medical Department already had a surgeon general (Col. Thomas Lawson) and after secession retained ninety-eight officers. Though Lawson died before the war was underway, he was replaced by Clement A. Finley, a senior army surgeon who had served since 1818.[42] There was thus a core of medical officers who had some military experience and institutionalized knowledge of how to manage army health (though this same group was not always the most broadminded). Yet the earliest volunteer regiments furnished their own regimental surgeons, most of whom were not properly examined. Because of the chaotic state of professional medicine some of these surgeons were scarcely qualified to wield a scalpel. Even when the government increased oversight of regimental surgeons in May of 1861, governors and colonels varied widely in their methods of securing medical personnel. Some demanded proper examinations, while others merely solicited confirmation from suspect medical boards. Justification for appointing men without medical degrees or training was that "scholarship" was not "the measure of practical ability." Thus surgeons' qualifications were spotty, and there was a drastic learning curve as the war progressed. Inexperience probably contributed greatly to the bungling inspection of new recruits that had led to unusually high rates of contagious disease in 1861.[43] It also led to improper management of camp sanitation, which would shortly come under civilian scrutiny.

The U.S. medical system, in fact, immediately garnered the attention of a group of high-profile citizens, who eventually cohered into a source of infrastructural strength beyond the traditional army network. As soon as there were U.S. soldiers in arms there were ladies' aid societies, who supported the troops with donations and homemade supplies. By April

1861, the New York ladies joined forces with Henry Whitney Bellows, an influential New York reformer and Unitarian pastor, and his acquaintance Dr. Elisha Harris to form the Women's Central Association of Relief (WCAR). WCAR meant to "collect and distribute information" in regards to the army's needs; to provide "lint, bandages, &c., in sustaining a central deposit of stores"; "to solicit and accept the aide of local associations"; and "especially to open a bureau for the examination and registration" of nurses. Unlike the military Medical Department, which had immediate fires to put out since droves of early recruits were sick, WCAR was able to take time to analyze the sources of mortality in the most recent world conflicts, including the Florida Seminole Wars, Mexican-American War, and the Crimean War. Its members determined that disease was by far the greater killer than battle wounds, despite the military's classical focus on surgery. They called attention to hygiene and environmental causation of disease, or specifically the effects of "change of climate and local situation."[44]

Shortly thereafter, Bellows pushed aside WCAR to advance the national U.S. Sanitary Commission, filling its board of managers with prominent male intellectuals, from Wall Street lawyer George Templeton Strong as treasurer to social leader and city planner Frederick Law Olmsted as secretary.[45] Considering the Commission's inherent critique of the military approach to medicine, it took intense lobbying to convince the War Department that the Commission would assist and not hamper the Medical Department. Commission historian Charles Janeway Stillé somberly remembered this period: "It is humiliating to record the utter inability [of the government] . . . to appreciate the best considered and most widely extended system of mitigating the horrors of war known in history and especially at a time when the existence of the Government was dependent upon the health and efficiency of that army which the appointment of a Sanitary Commission was designed to promote." President Lincoln finally permitted the "Commission of Inquiry and Advice in Respect of the Sanitary interests of the United States forces," though carefully limited in scope, on June 13, 1861.[46] Its first task in the field—dispatching inspectors to the eastern and western theaters to investigate camp conditions—was also one of its most contentious. Civilian inspectors were to walk among military encampments, recording information on soldiers' diets, water quality, clothing, quarters, hospitals, medical staff, the quantity and purity of medicines, and sanitary regulations—including ventilation, types of disinfectants, and overall cleanliness of the men and camps.[47]

The results of the inspections shocked commission members and prompted them to push the U.S. Medical Department toward vigorous reform in 1862. Commission members also slowly sought to expand their roles in fostering improved army health and morale. Secretary Olmsted himself had investigated the vicinity of Washington, D.C., and issued a December 1861 report to the U.S. secretary of war that would help to frame the restructuring of the Medical Department.[48] Olmsted wrote that an alarming number of men— "fifty-eight per cent of the regiments"— had not been adequately screened by surgeons before being enlisted. This oversight amounted to "the startling conclusion that fully fifty-three per cent. of the whole number [of the 1,620 soldiers from the Army of the Potomac discharged as unfit for service during the month of October] were thus discharged on account of disabilities that existed at and before their enlistment, and which any intelligent surgeon ought to have discovered on their inspection as recruits." Thus, future surgeons would have to be more adequately examined. Olmsted went on to state that "camp sites have been generally selected for military reasons alone, and with little if any regard to sanitary considerations," which threw increased scrutiny upon the priorities of generals. Tents, Olmsted continued, within camps were too close together and often overcrowded with poor ventilation, while those regiments with improperly situated or filthy privies yielded the sickest men. Here the implicit appraisal was that regimental officers were failing to enforce discipline. His next critique was less subtle. Olmsted denounced that "about eighty per cent" of the regimental officers "claimed that they gave systematic attention to the personal cleanliness of the men . . . [although] in very few instances—almost none—is this attention what it should be." He particularly cited dirty feet and, in 90 percent of the volunteers, dirty clothing. Further, officers had disregarded simple solutions for low morale, lacking recreational materials and open-air exercise. And finally, in confirmation of an old military paradigm, Olmsted's data showed that regular regiments exhibited better personal cleanliness and health than volunteer regiments.[49] This last point would reinforce a class bias against volunteer common soldiers that they not only lacked the training but the self-discipline required for good army health. While it was generally accurate that professional soldiers were more disciplined than volunteers, Olmsted's more important point was that improved discipline began with officer oversight.

Presented with a clear need for improvement, change to the U.S. military medical system occurred from within and without in early 1862. General-in-Chief George McClellan, for instance, had ordered regimental surgeons to examine their men to make up for initial neglect, and he punished the noncompliant.[50] More important, the Commission urged a medical reform bill through Congress. The bill replaced Surgeon General Finley, who was hostile toward the Commission, with William Alexander Hammond, whose impressive scholarship and army career on the frontier recommended him. It also called for a permanent corps of inspectors to investigate sanitation in hospitals, camps, and quarters, new hospital construction standards in the European pavilion style (which allowed for better ventilation and sanitation), an organized ambulance system under the Medical Department rather than the Quartermaster Department, and medical appointments based on merit rather than seniority.[51] The Commission additionally expanded its practices of contributing supplies and nurses, increasing interaction with soldiers, and began to offer new services, such as providing floating hospitals to transport and care for the sick and wounded on the Peninsula. The Commission's structures were integrated into the military system; the quartermaster's department provided it with transportation routes, steamers, and supply lines.[52] Further, the Commission inaugurated a paper campaign to educate inexperienced surgeons and officers, distributed up-to-date medical treatises on many of the diseases with supposed environmental origins—in effect, a portable library for field surgeons—and collected medical data on soldiers. Among statistics collected were "the effect[s] of climate, locality, and mode of life upon men."[53]

Over the course of 1862, Surgeon General Hammond proved a considerable asset to the Union military medical establishment. He proposed his own set of reforms, augmenting medical staff, raising the standards for the appointment of surgeons, establishing a graduate medical school in Washington to keep medical officers apprised of the latest scientific advances, and collecting medical data that would be incorporated into a new museum. Many of his proposals had to be approved by Congress, a slow process, meaning that the period of the two campaigns of this study was most often marked by critical decisions rather than tangible change.[54] Hammond did, however, move quickly on the issues within his power, such as releasing circulars to improve the flow of information regarding disease. For instance, the May 21, 1862, Circular No. 2 called for surgeons to give particular attention to "preventable diseases" in their monthly reports, such as keeping a precise catalogue of fever symptoms along with "an outline of the plans of treatment found most efficient with remarks on the location and sanitary condition of camps, or quarters, during the prevalence of these disorders." For dysentery and diarrhea it called for information on the "grade and treatment, with remarks on the character of the ration, and the modes of cooking," and for scurvy "observations on causation, and a statement of the means employed to procure exemption." In regards to respiratory diseases, surgeons were to look to environmental impetus "with remarks on the sheltering of the troops, and the atmospheric conditions."[55] In short, the orders addressed many of the problems the soldiers had already isolated in their accounts. In addition, Hammond replaced the ineffectual Peninsula medical director, Charles S. Tripler, with Jonathan Letterman. Letterman made important strides in medical evacuation, calling for "the consolidation of field hospitals at the division level, decentralization of medical control of ambulances to the regimental level, and centralization of medical control of ambulances at all levels."[56] Letterman's ambulance system, however, would only be in full effect for the battle of Antietam in September 1862 and would not become official U.S. Army policy until 1864.[57] All told, 1862 brought instability but also promise to the Union army medical system.

The Confederacy, meanwhile, had to construct a Medical Department from scratch. This was both handicap and advantage, the latter in that the War Department did not need to appease stodgy figures in the military bureaucracy and could therefore avoid frequent turnover in its top medical positions. The Confederate Medical Department of the regular army was established by the Provisional Congress in Montgomery, Alabama, on February 26, 1861, consisting of a surgeon general (briefly David C. DeLeon, followed by Samuel Preston Moore in July 1861, who held the position for the duration of the war), four surgeons, and six assistant surgeons. In March, May, and August, the department was expanded to authorize additional medical officers, though there remained a critical shortage of surgeons and assistant surgeons in 1862. Surgeon General Moore directed field and general hospitals for the first two years of the war, but medical directors of the armies and geographical departments also had some control over medical officers and hospitals within their regions.[58] This setup encumbered the movement of supplies and staff, contributing to an already critical supply problem. Indeed, until 1862, Confederate surgeons had to equip themselves, providing their own medicines.

At the same time, the Confederacy did not have the benefit of an organized civilian relief effort with the dimension of the U.S. Sanitary Commission. Individual ladies' aid societies provided homespun goods and services, while others civilians volunteered as doctors and nurses, but there was no central organization dedicated to civilian oversight of the military's Medical Department. Supervision would have to come from Congress and the War Department. Still, the ladies who contributed reaped praise for their scattered efforts. The *Staunton Spectator* remarked, "From the beginning of the war, they have been doing all that was within the sphere of their power to do for the comfort and relief of our soldiers. . . . When needed, they made with their own fair hands, though unused to toil, Caps, Jackets, Pants, Drawers, Shirts, Gloves and Socks for the soldiers. When sick, they ministered to their comfort and relief, by all the means which their sex knows so well how to employ." On June 6, it singled out the "Ladies' Soldiers' Aid Society for the Natural Bridge District," which had invited "one hundred of our wounded soldiers to make their houses their homes during their convalescence."[59]

As with health care in the Union, 1862 inaugurated a tide of change for the better in the Confederate medical system. Legislators passed a medical reorganization bill, though President Davis vetoed it because it failed to allow for additional medical officers and did not adequately specify the duties of the proposed infirmary corps that would be attached to each brigade. Surgeon General Moore, much like his Union counterpart, strove to build up a competent medical staff. He oversaw the implementation of examinations, organized the Association of Army and Navy Surgeons of the Confederate States by 1863, and eventually encouraged the publication of the *Confederate States Medical and Surgical Journal* in 1864–1865. While these advances had little influence over the events of 1862, Moore was a capable administrator and made quick strides in hospital construction, creating a network of Virginia hospitals linked by railroad. The surgeon general also consolidated Richmond hospitals and placed them on elevated ground near clean water to protect against swamp miasmas and filth, demonstrating attention to environmental management.[60] He also facilitated a growing relationship between the only Confederate medical college that remained intact during the war—the Medical College of Virginia—and the Confederacy's Medical Department. The college's location in Richmond, the capital, made it a prime hospital location as well as a training ground for Confederate doctors in need of war experience. Two classes of physicians matriculated per year, and graduates were immediately offered examinations for appointment in the Confederate army; it was only in the later years of the war that the benefits of having well-trained surgeons in the army bore fruit.[61] On the whole, because of its more limited resources the Confederacy was able to implement a less rigorous overhaul of medical infrastructures in 1862 than did the Union.

Despite the improving medical infrastructures on both sides, only some of the changes would have impacts on the two campaigns of this study. Eighteen sixty-two was early in the conflict, and mobilization—even the rapid mobilization that characterized the Civil War—took time. Because a democratic society required civilian dominance over the military, Congress had to approve major changes, while the respective War Departments, presidents, generals, and their officers quibbled over their implementation as components of a complex bureaucracy. U.S. Sanitary Commission officials tended to be most vocal in their critiques about the excruciatingly slow execution of reform. Olmsted grumbled from the Peninsula that he was "piecing out . . . the deficiencies of the Medical Department in respect to the accommodation for the sick," while the surgeon general and the Commission's President Bellows had become infected with the ineptitude of the War Department, or "made a little sick by the atmosphere of Washington."[62] From Bellows's perspective, he was trying, but Secretary of War Edwin M. Stanton stood in his way. When he approached the secretary, Stanton had not even read the April reform bill and became "very pale" and "angry" at the insinuation that he had dragged his feet: "The Government will act when it gets ready!" he allegedly spat at Bellows.[63] Bellows demurred, but still little happened. Meanwhile, medical personnel on the ground were left to navigate the continuing health crisis in the ranks, which had evolved into a much larger problem than rescuing green soldiers from contagious diseases.

THE LIMITS OF OFFICIAL CARE

The soldiers tended to blame shortcomings of the inchoate medical system on individuals, and it indeed fell to military commanders, officers, surgeons, and medical staff to implement sorely needed change. The higher up the chain of command, the more an individual's decision could impact an army, and yet soldier health was a complex problem that evaded simple top-down solutions, especially when the keenest scientific minds of the age disagreed about disease causation and treatment. Hazy understanding along with the well-established biases associated with volunteer soldiers contributed to a deepening fatalism among those in charge of soldier health, evident particularly among surgeons. As soldiers died of disease, individuals deflected responsibility, which was easy to do considering they were involved in an expansive bureaucracy. Focusing on surgery rather than sickness proved a far more satisfying endeavor for military and medical staff, hence the reform focus on improving ambulance evacuation from the battlefield. Wounds had clear remedies and smacked of sacrifice in battle, while disease made everyone look incompetent. As Confederate surgeon William Taylor put it, "It was on the battlefield that the assistant surgeon was in his own sphere, for it was the method of our service for him to be with the troops when they were in action. Here he did his strenuous work."[64]

Atop the chain of command, military commanders had to take ultimate responsibility for the survival of their men. From commanders' perspectives a number of factors contributed to their inability to alleviate soldier suffering in 1862, though they did recognize that environment played some role in poor health and deteriorating morale. A considerable complaint in 1862, particularly in the Shenandoah Valley, was lack of supplies. A dearth of tents and clothes exposed soldiers unnecessarily to the elements, insufficient rations weakened troops' bodies, and limited medications and hospitals meant that those who inevitably fell ill faced deficient care. Union general John C. Frémont provides an especially instructive example of how a general of eminent experience in wartime environments could consider himself utterly unequal to the task of protecting his army's health. "The Pathfinder," who had served as a junior officer in the Army Corps of Engineers from 1842–1853 in five expeditions in the American West, surviving blizzards, frostbite, and starvation, was stunned by the "inclemencies of a spring seldom paralleled for severity in the history of the Virginia Valley."[65] Thanks to extreme supply shortages, he lamented that "as late as April 19, that so illy provided in other respects were the coming reenforcements that thirty-eight days had been passed by them without tents or other shelter." According to the Frémont, the root of supply paucity was complex: a "want of funds" in the quartermaster's department, farmers' refusal to submit their food along Union supply lines, and the impassability of the water-laden roads for carriages. He knew resultant exposure was compounding a dire health situation. "For last three days the weather has been terrible; constant blinding storm of snow, mixed with rain, which freezes to trees and limbs to extent as to bend and break them. . . . Men suffering."[66] And thus, as the privation and environmental misery wore on through May and June, he was hardly surprised at the near dissolution of the ranks, indicating mass demoralization: "demonstrations among the men, amounting to almost open mutiny."[67] With less than one full ration left to issue, "upward of 1,000 [sick soldiers] were now at Mount Jackson." Further, "the hospitals were full, and I was deficient in the necessary medicines, as well as the requisite number of surgeons to give attendance." In his helplessness, the general expressed typical class-based admiration for his men's ability to endure what were fast becoming insurmountable odds. "The heroism, the uncomplaining patience, with which the soldiers of my command endured the starvation and other bodily sufferings of their extended marches, added to their never-failing alacrity for duty against the enemy, entitle them to my gratitude and respect."[68] In short, Frémont's army was experiencing logistical meltdown, and his men were virtually on their own to make the best of a bleak situation.[69]

While the commanding general had to give an account for his disease casualties and the state of his army's morale, technically the medical director was supposed to oversee health matters. What happened after he made recommendations he could not necessarily control because of the nature of chain of command. In Frémont's area, the Union medical director was George Cooper Suckley, who also had considerable experience managing war environments as a former army doctor out west. He had participated in the Stevens' Survey for a Northern Pacific railroad route in 1853, served in the Northwest Indian wars of 1854–58, and traveled in an 1859 overland expedition to Utah, becoming a published naturalist along the way.[70] His spring 1862 attempts to call attention to soldier health read as though from a desperate man. For instance, "In the name of humanity I respectfully call the earnest attention of the commanding general to the sanitary condition of the division under the command of Brigadier-General Blenker. . . . I would state that nearly 200 men of Blenker's division are left behind in hospitals or straggling in our rear. There are about 200 more sick in this encampment." Suckley lacked ambulances for transporting the sick, and for the few carriages he had, his horses were no more than "skeletons." In Blenker's whole division there was "but one hospital tent," most of the medical supplies had been abandoned in haste, and the men themselves were "weary and haggard" with "stragglers . . . coming in until after dark, most of them weary and foot-sore, and many sick." Knowing that requesting supplies was an uphill struggle, Suckley suggested the only remedy that did not require them: twenty-four hours rest.[71]

It was not that the U.S. War Department was ignoring the deplorable state of affairs in the Shenandoah Valley. Peter H. Watson, the assistant secretary of war, wrote on May 27 to Secretary Stanton that troops near Harpers Ferry "have no intrenching tools, neither have they shelter or other tents sufficient for their protection from the dews, which are heavy, and exposures to which generate miasmatic diseases of a very obstinate and malignant type."[72] In other words, those in Washington comprehended the effects the environment of war were having on their unprotected troops, but military prerogatives—namely, balancing the defense of Washington, the more important Peninsula campaign for Richmond, and the three armies in the Valley—prevented swift rectification of the Valley logistical logjam. Even the quartermaster general was distracted trying to help Lincoln direct military strategy.[73]

While Frémont's situation demonstrates that supplies crucially under-pinned the medical system, Stonewall Jackson's command style ignited its own set of drawbacks and some benefits to the health of Confederate troops in the Valley. Jackson earned a reputation for being "rather indifferent to the comfort of his troops, & they are broken down very fast."[74] Viewed through the eyes of Confederate regimental surgeons, it is apparent that Jackson could be inflexible in accommodating medical needs that interfered with his strategic goals. For instance, William R. Whitehead, a surgeon with former experience in the Crimean, noted that despite "a rigid police" of his 44th Virginia's encampment on the western slope of the Alleghenies, "its soil after a few weeks became foul and numerous cases of fever occurred, followed by a number of deaths." He removed some of the sick "to the top of the Alleghany Mountains," where he believed they recovered from change of air and the fresh milk of local dairy, but he also requested that the camp be moved "a short distance away" to preserve the health of the remaining troops. His request was denied, because the current camp was "a strategic position." Yet "no enemy appeared, and we remained in the very limited area that our encampment occupied, with its regular streets of tents, losing from typhoid fever and other diseases, more men than the casualties of a battle might have occasioned." While Whitehead was hampered by the rigidity of his superiors, he tempered his disapproval with later praise for the quick pace of campaign. "Later in the war Gen'l T.J. Jackson . . . kept us almost constantly on the march and changing camp, which contributed to the efficiency, and general health of his army."[75] Being on the move meant the armies were less likely to foul the water and soil with encampment. One drawback of rapidity was that it wore down the troops and increased their exposure, ultimately becoming a major problem when Jackson's men were called to the Peninsula to reinforce Lee. Many of Jackson's foot soldiers would be too fatigued to effectively participate, leading to a spike in straggling and desertion. For the duration of the Valley campaign, both Jackson's and his medical director Hunter McGuire's reports on soldier health would focus on the wounded rather than the sick, betraying a command-level bias toward celebrating those who had sacrificed in combat and overlooking (or even scrutinizing) those who were sick. But McGuire did improve the infirmary corps in the spring of 1862, in which roughly thirty unfit men were assigned simple nursing duties for the wounded and sick.[76]

Those managing health on the Peninsula faced a less dire supply situation, if still a shortage of available hospital space.[77] Yet the stagnant pace of the campaign made preventing sickness in the camps difficult and made the Union's General McClellan, in particular, defensive of his strategic choices. He warned President Lincoln in May of 1862, "Delays on my part will be dangerous. I fear sickness and demoralization. This region is unhealthy for Northern men, and, unless kept moving, I fear that our soldiers may become discouraged. At present our numbers are weakening from disease, but our men remain in good heart."[78] His surgeons agreed with him. In May, Union surgeon Castleman wrote, "We are now in an intensely malarious region, with the sun's scorching rays pouring on us, and our men coming down by scores daily. We have been nearly twelve months in the field, have fought but one battle, and I fear that General McClellan's plan, to win by delay, without a fight, is poor economy of human life."[79] A month later, Union surgeon William M. Smith lamented, "One of the largest, best and most munificently appointed armies ever led into battle has been wasted in the poisonous swamps of the Peninsula."[80] And yet as McClellan watched the rivers swell from rain and his army deteriorate from illness, he fixated mainly upon acquiring more troops from Washington.

It was not that McClellan had not tried to get to the bottom of what ailed his army. The general himself had suffered from typhoid fever in the winter, and in December 1861 he had ordered a "fever board" to investigate hospital conditions and question medical officers about the causes of the fevers plaguing the army. Little insight was gleaned, however, as the board pronounced that rampant typhoid fever resulted from blood poisoning, the very characterization of disease causation from which contemporary medicine was retreating.[81] The diagnosis did not point to a need for increased sanitation or environmental management and, therefore, did not help McClellan solve the increasing fever epidemic once the Peninsula campaign commenced. By June, when Secretary Stanton lambasted McClellan over a number of health concerns, including underutilizing hospital space and failing to provide the troops with fresh water, McClellan retorted that "the care of our sick & wounded has tasked the unremitted energies of the whole medical corps in this army as well as occupied a great share of my attention from other important duties & I feel conscious that everything has been done for their comfort that human efforts could accomplish."[82] The comment betrayed his impatience with the complexity of army health. He blamed his inaction and the widespread illness on "infamous" weather, the treacherous rise of the Chickahominy River, and the resulting fact that his men had to work "night and day up to their waists in water. . . . The whole face of the country is a perfect bog."[83] When it ceased raining McClellan realized the heat was equally detrimental: "We are to have another very hot day, I fancy; no air stirring, and the atmosphere close and murky. I don't wish to spend the summer on the banks of this river; we will fry or bake!"[84] In short, environmental factors evidently contributed to poor health, but what was a commander to do? The waterlogged expanse of Peninsula separated the Army of the Potomac from the Confederacy's capital and had to be endured. The general may have been slow, but he also was dealt a supremely sickly and environmentally challenging location in summer.[85]

McClellan did have a loyal medical director, Charles Tripler, to assist, but Tripler became consumed by the same power struggles distracting McClellan. Early on, Tripler went around the surgeon general and secretary of war to "do McClellan's bidding," making him unpopular in the War Department and contributing to his eventual removal in July.[86] Yet this was hardly Tripler's main distraction. He also faced significant supply problems and bureaucratic sluggishness. The Army of the Potomac's location on a peninsula, surrounded by water, meant Tripler had to be supplied by ship and look to floating hospitals for bed space, requiring constant negotiating with the U.S. Navy and Sanitary Commission. His ideas for improving health were logical enough, if sometimes unimaginative in execution. For instance, supposing that swamp miasmas were the major cause of illness in the ranks, Tripler ordered the hospitals to slightly higher ground at White House Landing on the Pamunkey, Fort Monroe, and Yorktown. But this did not prevent men from becoming ill and occupying the beds. Though Tripler answered to McClellan, he could not always convince command that health needs ought to influence military strategy. In one example, Tripler acknowledged that "the greatest proportion [of typhoid fever] occurred in Keyes' corps, on our left. The country occupied by him was the worst on the Peninsula, and, in addition to that, one of his divisions was composed of our newest troops," but nothing came of his concern.[87] The medical director also had difficulty implementing remedies for the emerging scurvy problem, though his medical advice was sound. On June 15, Tripler reported: "I have ordered a supply of lemons and cream of tartar from White House to Sumner's corps . . . and desiccated vegetables [should] be immediately ordered to be issued as parts of the daily rations, and that the commanding officers should be charged with the duty of seeing them daily and properly used."[88] But he admitted that the men hated desiccated vegetables. As soldier Abner Small explained, they were "some kind of vegetable compound in portable form . . . in sheets like pressed hops. . . . What in Heavens name it was composed of, none of us ever discovered." In order to cook the substance, a man would "break off a piece as large as a boot top, put it in a kettle of water, and stir it with the handle of a hospital broom. When the stuff was fully dissolved, the water would remind one of a dirty brook with all the dead leaves floating around promiscuously."[89] Tripler's plan was thus untenable. Reports of scurvy skyrocketed by the time Tripler was removed from his post.

By the end of his tenure, Tripler appeared to have lost touch with the severity of the health crisis in the Army of the Potomac. Though official estimates placed the sick rolls at around thirty percent of forces, with diarrhea and dysentery exploding into a veritable epidemic, Tripler reported the following: "During this campaign the army was favored with excellent health. No epidemic diseases appeared. Those scourges of modern armies—dysentery, typhus, cholera—were almost unknown." He continued, "We had some typhoid fever and more malarial fever, but even these never prevailed to such an extent as to create any alarm. The sick reports were sometimes larger than we cared to have them, but the great majority of the cases reported were such as did not threaten life or permanent disability." But the truly incongruous claim was this: "My recollection is that the whole sick report never exceeded 8 per cent. . . . The Army of the Potomac must be conceded to have been the most healthy army in the service of the United States."[90] When pressed to explain the disease casualties, Tripler blamed his inferiors, the surgeons beneath him, for their incompetence.[91]

When newly appointed U.S. Surgeon General Hammond replaced Tripler with Jonathan Letterman, the new medical director for the Army of the Potomac made strides in managing army health that would pay off over time. While his most important improvements addressed the evacuation of the wounded by ambulance corps, he did curb the scurvy epidemic, addressed mental health, and strove to improve camp conditions.[92] When Letterman arrived on the Peninsula, he immediately recorded his observations on the environmental origins of disease with considerable optimism. "The diseases prevailing in our army are generally of a mild type and are not increasing. Their chief causes are, in my opinion, the want of proper food (and that improperly prepared), exposure to the malaria of swamps and the inclemencies of the weather, excessive fatigue, and want of natural rest, combined with great excitement of several days' duration, and the exhaustion consequent thereon." Perhaps his composure stemmed from the fact that he had plans for action. His detailed instructions to the officers included that "wells be dug as deep as the water will permit; that the troops be provided with tents or other shelter to protect them from the sun and rain, which shall be raised daily and struck once a week and placed upon new ground . . . that the men be required to cut pine tops, spread them thickly in their tents, and not sleep on the ground; that camps be formed not in the woods but at a short distance from them, where a free circulation of pure air can be procured, and where the ground has been exposed to the sun and air to such an extent as to vitiate the noxious exhalations from damp ground saturated with emanations from the human body and from the decaying vegetation."[93] His suggestions, which mitigated exposure to bad weather, water, and air, reflected the best medical knowledge of the time and displayed a new commitment to prevention along the lines of reforms the U.S. Sanitary Commission was seeking.

While many of Letterman's proposals would take time to execute given that they relied upon officer cooperation, he made immediate progress in the area of nutrition, unlike his predecessor. He quickly oversaw the distribution of fresh vegetables, fruit, and fresh bread as anti-scorbutics— more palatable than desiccated vegetables—after receiving reports of an alarming number of scurvy cases. In response he saw success: "The beneficial effects of this treatment soon became perceptible on the health of the men, and when we left Harrison's Landing scurvy had disappeared from the Army of the Potomac." It is clear from other accounts that it took longer for some regiments to receive the anti-scorbutics than others but that eventually the cases of scurvy did abate.[94] Letterman also issued orders for improved cooking, heralding the health benefits of soup: "The importance of soup as a diet for troops is not sufficiently appreciated except by veteran soldiers, those of experience in the field."[95] Poor cooking was a known cause of diarrhea, and though unbeknownst to contemporaries, encouraging the boiling of ingredients in soup effectively eradicated the bacteria and amoebae behind the problem.

Letterman likewise took a comprehensive approach to morale. For instance, he noted the correlation between poor physical and mental health and their connections with environmental conditions. "Scurvy," he observed, "was not due merely to the want of vegetables, but also to exposure to cold and wet, working and sleeping in the mud and rain, and to the inexperience of these troops in taking proper care of themselves under difficult circumstances." He further concluded, "This disease is not to be dreaded merely by the numbers it sends upon the reports of the sick. It goes much further, and the causes which give rise to it undermine the strength, depress the spirits, take away the energy, courage, and elasticity of those who do not report themselves sick, and yet their energy, their powers of endurance, and their willingness to undergo hardship are in a great degree gone, and they know not why." In short, "it had affected the fighting powers of the army."[96] Thus eradicating scurvy would improve army morale. Letterman also worked to keep the sick nearby their units rather than remove them from their comrades, increasing spirits. And yet, despite these significant improvements, when the army gathered at Harrison's Landing in July and August, its condition remained dire. Letterman worried that his men were mentally and physically weak even before they reached Harrison's Landing because of "the want of proper nourishment, the poisonous exhalations from the streams and swamps of the Peninsula, the labor undergone, and the anxiety felt."[97]

On the one hand, the Confederates faced a similar problem of stagnancy and swamps on the Peninsula, though they did enjoy a slight advantage of occupying the higher ground.[98] As Confederate surgeon Spencer G. Welch explained, environment remained taxing for them: "All the tents have been taken away from the men, and that, together with the change of climate from the coast of South Carolina to this place, has caused much sickness in our regiment."[99] On the other hand, Confederates suffered from a problem unique to their country: a critical paucity of quinine to combat the widespread malaria raging through the swamps of the Peninsula.[100] As with many of the other generals commanding armies, Johnston, a Virginian and West Pointer of diverse and considerable military experience, well understood the environmental influence on health.[101] In his memoirs, he even reflected, "Those who have seen large bodies of new troops know that they are sickly in all climates. . . . The troops of the Army of the Shenandoah suffered as much in the healthy climate of the Valley as they and others did at Centreville and Fairfax County."[102] His knowledge apparently grew into fatalism when it came to counteracting the sickly environment he observed, as there is little evidence to show he acted upon his wisdom.[103]

Johnston's successor, Lee, was more proactive in improving soldier discipline, which was, perhaps, the simplest way for command to address the health crisis. As historian Joseph Glatthaar has pointed out, Lee followed up concern with action, urging improved sanitation and cooking habits among his men.[104] Yet Lee had inherited difficulties that he could not amend during the Seven Days campaign. A crippling combination of poor maps and unreliable guides made it difficult to plot out camp organization, and a quickly advancing front made it difficult for supply trains to provide for the men. The soldiers took what they could from Union troops, but it was never enough.[105] Though Lee was more aggressive at moving his troops than Johnston, he made leadership errors early in his command that contributed to operational inefficiency. He attempted to direct too many details personally and often issued overly complex orders to his officers, engendering confusion in the chain of command. Disorder limited his initiatives to improve health.[106] And yet Lee was a disciplinarian who believed in taking the time necessary to teach green soldiers to acclimate to soldier life. In mid-August, he pondered reorganizing and moving his army as the campaign on the Peninsula came to a close. On August 14, he wrote Jefferson Davis: "The two [new] N.C. regts: from Salisbury & Lynchburg are ordered to D. H. Hill. . . . I thought they would do better then, having not yet been in the field & give them a better opportunity for instruction & to pass through the camp diseases."[107]

The Army of Northern Virginia did not experience the same tumultuous turnover in medical leadership on the Peninsula as did the Army of the Potomac, but Lee's medical director, Lafayette Guild, much like Jackson's Valley medical director Hunter McGuire, appeared far more preoccupied with battle wounds. Appointed just before the Seven Days campaign, Guild would order division medical wagons to stock extra blankets, clothes, vegetables, and tea just before an imminent battle. He explained that the wounded would need new clothing and careful attention, though he did not suggest the same benefits for the sick. Indeed, Guild was sluggish at addressing even scurvy. Though Confederate ration ledgers show the addition of fruits and vegetables in the summer of 1862, Guild did not personally address the problem until early 1863. He then noted a "tendency to scorbutus throughout the whole" Army of Northern Virginia and warned about the need for an increase in vegetables.[108]

While commanders and medical directors were most influential in shaping health policy and determining the location of armies, regimental officers were responsible for enforcing discipline, which critically shaped the way the soldiers experienced the environment of war. Men looked to their officers as examples and for orders regarding camp layout, camp maintenance, and personal hygiene. Commission secretary Olmsted had critiqued officers in his December report for failing to keep their men clean, and the Commission inspection returns from the early part of 1862 corroborated his concern. The reports confirmed that the healthiest camps were those in which regimental officers took responsibility for inspecting the kitchens, latrines, and tents of their men, while unhealthy camps featured trash piled in the streets, men dropping their trousers wherever they pleased, and negligent officers.[109] In some cases those officers who were inexperienced volunteers themselves did not know or appreciate the importance of army regulations. In other cases, much to the frustration of Sanitary Commission members, some officers resented playing "chambermaid" to the men.[110]

While officers and medical directors passed responsibility back and forth, regimental surgeons and hospital staffers ultimately had to treat the sick men and argued their own reasons for what they acknowledged was inadequate care. Olmsted, as usual, had choice words for what he characterized as the surgeons' neglect. He claimed surgeons had laid the sick and wounded "in tiers in the muddy streets" of Yorktown and "a hundred sick had been left . . . in the rain, without attendance or food, to die.'"[111] Surgeons, alternately, explained that they had not enough hospitals, supplies, or staff to attend to the vast numbers of ailing men. For instance, when Chaplain Twichell found eighteen men lying out in plain air on the Peninsula, suffering from typhoid, five "dying," some "insensible, others raving," and "none of them [with] their clothes off," he was determined to find the surgeon and make him give an account for such suffering. "We found the Surgeon in charge, who appeared to be a man of energy and ability. He told a sad story of much to do, with nothing to do it with and noone to help."[112] Confederate surgeon E. A. Craighill explained a similar situation, as he helplessly observed a new brigade of Georgians quickly demolished from measles, pneumonia, and diarrhea. They "had no comforts or hospital accommodations for the poor fellows, not even tents . . . and their suffering was intense."[113] But this is not to say that some surgeons did not confirm episodes of neglect. Castleman complained bitterly in his diary about "surgeons, whose only notoriety consists in their ability to stand up under the greatest amount of whisky; and also against their re-appointing surgeons under the same influence who, after examination, have been mustered out of the service for incompetency. Under such appointments humanity is shocked, and a true and zealous army of patriots dwindle rapidly into a mass of mal-contents."[114]

Surgeons also balked at their subservience to the higher ranks, who, as has been outlined, navigated their own competing interests in military bureaucracy. Most Civil War surgeons were, after all, volunteers themselves and not used to taking orders, especially when it came to saving lives. Confederate surgeon Aristides Monteiro became searingly cynical when looking back on 1862 in his memoirs. "May the angels and ministers of grace, watch and defend a brave army against the diabolical machinery of organic military medicine. . . . Unfortunately, in military medicine, the fool and the charlatan is powerful if he has procured a commission through the pusillanimous influence of nepotism." Even the best intentioned would be corrupted by the system. "Should a surgeon be so indiscrete as to manifest any human feeling or sympathy for the sick or wounded under his care, he would surely be reprimanded for the kindness of his heart. To please the head of the department, surgeons must be cruel, stern, severe; and above all things, stupid, submissive, and sycophantic."[115] Such harsh words probably had most to do with Monteiro's feelings of helplessness.

Not only did superiors fail to listen to health recommendations when military necessity dictated otherwise, but surgeons were part of a system that did not foster good relationships between patient and doctor. As Castleman explained, promotion could be painful when it meant removal from the men who were "intimate personal friends" and the sons of "my neighbors and friends" to a distant hospital. On June 5, Castleman called on Tripler, the Peninsula medical director, "and stated in the strongest language I could command, my wishes to be with my regiment . . . who looked to me for aid and comfort in the time of trial, and I would like to be present, even if only long enough to receive their dying messages." Tripler was unmoved. *"I did not get the permission."*[116] Surgeon Jonah F. Dyer of the 19th Massachusetts pointed out that it was also difficult for doctors to follow up with patients given the nature of military life: "Sick and wounded are as soon as possible transferred to general hospital, and as regimental surgeons are employed principally in the field, they rarely see their patients but a few times."[117] He lamented the resultant lack of personal contact and long-term care, but this reality also meant that doctors would never learn if their patients recovered based on their treatments. It was thus difficult for surgeons to untangle the persistent mysteries shrouding disease.

Further, the nature of the military hierarchy sometimes bred trifling disputes that ensnared surgeons. Castleman related an anecdote in which his medical staff presented him with a sword as a token of their gratitude for his service. What began as a gesture of kindness precipitated a display of "petty tyranny" on the parts of his superiors, who reprimanded and then removed his staff for improper conduct, replacing them with incompetents. Castleman reacted bitterly on March 6: "There is not a man amongst [the new staff] who can make a toast or broil a chicken; yet the sick must depend on them for all their cooking. Not one has ever dispensed a dose of medicine, and yet I must depend on them for this duty. It is a dreadful thought to me that I must go to the battle field with the set which is now around me." Indeed, their ineptitude sprang from the fact that they were not nurses at all, but "half of them are applicants for discharge on the ground of disability, yet they are sent to me to work over the sick, night and day, and to carry the wounded from the battle field." The results of the general's "vindictive meddling with the Medical Department" were as Castleman predicted. On March 13, "The druggist knew not one medicine from another, and to-day three men are poisoned by a mistake in dispensing medicines. One of them is already dead; the other two suffering severely, though I have hopes that they may yet be saved." In a sad twist, the druggist even managed to poison himself, "taking pills of Unguentum—blue mercurial ointment—instead of blue pill, which had been prescribed for him." The preparation contained about twenty percent mercury, yet the man survived for the time being. Castleman contemptuously labeled the situation proof of the "fatherly care which our General is manifesting towards the soldiers under his command."[118]

Dyer reported several similar stories in which his superiors' personal agendas blocked his ability to administer quality care. On April 10, 1862, in camp near Yorktown, Dyer derided General McClellan for ordering a rapid advance, which precipitated mass discarding of tents. For a military imperative Dyer may have conceded, but this was a typical McClellan flourish; the general advanced his army just far enough to lose the tents but not confront the enemy. The result, according to Dyer, was a crisis of exposure. Dyer was also one of the first to identify the scurvy outbreak among Union ranks on the Peninsula. He mentioned the problem on June 14, 1862: "Several cases of scurvy have occurred in our brigade, a few in our regiment. This is owing to the want of fresh vegetables. We have had potatoes issued as a ration but once since we came on the Peninsula, and even vinegar but seldom." When he tried to report the need for issuing vegetables to the ranks, headquarters dismissed him. "The troops should not have scurvy. Their rations are plentiful and good. Therefore scurvy does not exist," said his supervisor. After more solicitation, headquarters finally sent a surgeon down to examine the men who confirmed the cases. Though even the newspapers reported on the scurvy epidemic and assured civilians that vegetables would be administered shortly, Dyer's regiment saw no sign of the improved rations for weeks.[119]

Many surgeons also freely admitted that they did not have the expertise or supplies to be effective caregivers. As Confederate surgeon William Taylor put it, during sick call in the morning "diagnosis was rapidly made, usually by intuition, and treatment was with such drugs as we chanced to have in the knap-sack and were handiest to obtain." For instance, one day he had a ball of blue mass in one pocket and a ball of opium in the other. He asked the soldiers how their bowels fared; if they had diarrhea he would give them opium, and if they were constipated he would administer the blue mass.[120] The process of sick call could be rushed or chaotic, making it difficult for surgeons to adequately assess symptoms even if they did recognize them.

Union surgeons were not without support in their difficult task to provide soldiers with care within the military system. As mentioned, the U.S. Sanitary Commission assembled and distributed a portable library, intended to outline the most current knowledge about disease and surgery. While providing an advantage for those physicians separated from their medical books, the knowledge the treatises presented was sometimes perplexingly contradictory. After all, there was a great diversity of medical opinions at the time, and the Commission assembled a pool of doctors to author the pamphlets. For instance, the treatises on "fevers," a popular topic for those stationed on the Peninsula, were particularly dense. There were many categories of fever, including typhoid, malaria, typhoid-malaria, typhus, irritative, intermittent, remittent, congestive, and other possible incarnations. Malarial fevers (and sometimes typhoid) were associated with swamp miasmas, dense foliage, coastal areas, and heat and humidity, while typhoid (and, confusingly at times, typhus, a completely unrelated parasitic disease usually transmitted by lice) was often termed "camp fever." Typhoid was linked to blood poisoning from overcrowding, poor hygiene, overexertion, and unhealthy air in hospitals and ships, but it could also have a mental origin in "anxiety, fatigue, want, deprivation, and misery." The cures for fever were as numerous as the fevers themselves, ranging from quinine to improving hygiene to relocating the patient to healthier air.[121]

The pamphlets' descriptions of diarrhea and dysentery were equally diverse. They were most often associated with exposure, swampy and miasmatic locations, the heat of summer and fall, neglect of proper sanitation, and typhoid.[122] Treatments ranged from opium to, appallingly, laxatives. Even scurvy, a relatively simple disease, was presented in a convoluted manner. The authors suggested scurvy could be from any of three origins: (1) physical and environmental—dark, cold, moisture, impure air, and lack of exercise; (2) moral—nostalgia, characterized by "despondency of mind," "mental depression," and anxiety; and (3) dietetic—the "deprivation of succulent vegetable food," as well as lack of fresh meat or sameness of diet. While the third alleged cause hinted at the truth—a lack of vitamin C— some doctors insisted that all three categories had to be present to incite disease. Treatments, unsurprisingly, varied to address the multiple causations, but vegetables—particularly citrus and potatoes—fresh air, leisure games, and reduced exposure were among prescriptions.[123]

It is no wonder that doctors, some of whom were not yet qualified to practice, were confused and incapable of applying successful treatment to the common diseases they encountered. They often tried to emphasize environmental management, such as cleanliness or change of location, but they could only work within the physical parameters presented them. Thomas F. Wood, an assistant surgeon from North Carolina, worked to control the indoor environment by directing the six nurses under his care to keep the hospital "scrupulously clean." He wrote, "It was scoured with a mop every morning, and dry scoured every afternoon. The floors were very white, although it was hard to keep the soldiers habitually in mind of clean habits."[124] Surgeon William M. Smith of the 85th New York had to be away from his regiment due to his own illness, and when he returned he was dismayed to find them in an unhealthy camp location. "I find the regiment encamped in a dense wood, in very low, wet ground," he noted on July 14. The men were pleased to see him return, especially because he immediately exerted his influence upon the commander to move camp. "We removed from our camp yesterday morning to a much more pleasant and healthy camp." But Smith revealed that this change had not been easily won: "No persuasion of the colonel could induce Gen. Wessells to give leave for the regiment to occupy [this] ground. And only after I made an official order to secure the health of the regiment would he yield; and then, rather ungracefully."[125] Dyer had a similar victory with change of location: "We are now about a mile from the river, a little out of the mud and alongside a small stream where the men can wash."[126]

Finally, surgeons often struggled to impart reasonable care to the soldiers, because they themselves were very sick. Though they were officers who had superior access to shelter, food, and medical supplies, they, too, had to undergo seasoning and were exposed to the sickly environment of war. John G. Perry, an assistant surgeon from Massachusetts, complained on August 1, "My cottage is full, in fact the whole hospital is crowded, and I am tired out, having no relief whatever from steady, close confinement." Immediately after Perry penned those words he was gripped by crippling illness and had to return home. He did not rejoin the army until April 11, 1863, after taking a hiatus to pass his medical board exams and marry his sweetheart.[127] Surgeon Smith, of the 85th New York, was nearly dead with exhaustion by June. "I left camp this P.M. (about 3 o'clock) for a few days rest from the toil which I have for several months past undergone without an hours rest. My health has come to imperatively demand it. For many years, I have not been so entirely sick and never as worn out as now."[128] Castleman watched first his fellow staff grow ill, and he himself followed shortly thereafter: "I am very hard worked just now. The Brigade Surgeon is sick, and I being the ranking Surgeon in the Brigade, have his duties to perform." But the situation was even worse than that: "In addition, I have charge, at present, of a large share of the Hospital of the 49th Regiment Penn. Vols., the Surgeon being very ill. That regiment is in dreadful condition. Very many of them are sick, and of very grave diseases." Further, his assistant had been suspended. "From altogether I am much worn down, and need rest." Castleman fell ill in March. "For three nights I have not slept, and last night I had an attack of cholera morbus. This morning, being sick and worn out, I asked permission to return to Vienna. . . . Permission was denied me."[129] If the surgeons were not allowed to attend to their own health, then soldiers had little hope of receiving suitable care.

Continuing with Castleman's story, it becomes evident how sick surgeons led to neglected men. After scarcely recovering from his illness on May 26, Castleman reported to the Liberty Hall Hospital, where 400 ill soldiers were crowded into one house and its stables, "alive with vermin—chicken houses, the stench of which would sicken a well man, on the ground, exposed alternately to beating rain and the rays of the scorching sun." He learned from the men that this was the third day during which they had lain without food, "or without any one to look after them, except as they could mutually aid each other." The men reeled with typhus, scurvy, diarrhea, and dysentery. As the doctor aptly put it, "To pitch what few tents I have, and to get as many as I can under shelter, I have before me, in the organization of this hospital, a Herculean task for a man not quite recovered from a spell of sickness. But what I can, I will do."[130]

All in all, those most responsible for administering care within the military systems believed their hands tied by a range of circumstances beyond their control. Someone else was always in charge of a critical component of care—be it supplies or location—while everyone served different priorities. Military commanders had to answer to their government and the populace by producing battlefield victories, and managing health was an unpleasant distraction. Surgeons usually believed their first responsibility was healing the soldiers but often could not act upon this concern. The result was a health crisis larger than the medical directors were willing to admit.

CIVILIAN PERSPECTIVES ON SOLDIER SICKNESS

If surgeons struggled to accommodate the sick, often blaming military hierarchy and the systems of which they were a part, at the end of the day blame circled back around to common soldiers as befit the cultural milieu. Civilians propagated a pervasive bias in the newspapers that linked army sickness to individual soldier behavior, while emphasizing the heroism of the Medical Departments and health care workers. Widespread disapproval of soldier behavior was born in part of the bias against volunteer soldiers, which had well-established historical antecedents. It was also fueled by reform movement zeal that linked poor health to a lack of self-control, reinforced by Second Great Awakening religiosity. Soldiers had to look no further than the daily news to realize that sympathy for their suffering only went so far.

Many of the reporters stressed the role a soldier's juvenile dietary preferences played in his poor bowel health. As the *Valley Spirit* put it, "The unfavorable influences of the Sutlers on the health of the men has already been referred to, and the free use of their pies, raisins, nuts, cheese, and similar indigestibles, doubtless cause much of the sickness and mortality among the men." In other words, the soldiers failed to spend their meager earnings in wise ways. Those who were sick in the ranks were "the greatest offenders in this respect. Their illness seemed to make some of them more like children than soldiers, and their morbid cravings for improper food could scarcely be restrained."[131] Infantilizing the soldiers—some of whom were, in fact, just teenagers—was failing to take into account the complete picture. The men missed home, which the so-called delicacies recalled to mind; they were often underfed and therefore hungry; and they were critically deprived of fruits and vegetables. This is not to say that non-regulation food was never suspect, as Private Fletcher discovered when he purchased from a peddler a sausage laden with cat bones.[132] Also subject to critique in the newspapers was the food sent from loved ones at home to the warfront. One anonymous corporal from the 77th Pennsylvania wrote the *Valley Spirit*, "We of course do not fare as well in regard to delicacies from our friends as we would if encamped near home, which I presume is better for us, as I have noticed whenever the boys have received boxes from home they are apt to get on the sick list."[133] Resisting such temptations appeared to the public to indicate that a soldier had been properly socialized into the army.

Besides warnings about proper diet, newspapers also drew attention to the general lack of discipline in the volunteer units. The Mexican-American War had proven that the professional army had a distinct advantage over the volunteer army, and impeccable discipline translated to better health. Thus the *Chicago Tribune* honed in on the familiar topic. "The per cent of sickness among the volunteers of the army, is greater than among the regulars. This is owing mainly to slackness of discipline."[134] In another example, a Union report praised that "with the improved discipline of the army, many of the officers are learning the first great lesson of military life, that it is their duty to take care of their men, not merely to command them. In the true spirit of the Christian soldier, many of the colonels now devote themselves not only to the drill, but to the sanitary condition of the men, and especially to the welfare of their sick."[135] This second report at least acknowledged the role officers played in fostering discipline, rather than focusing all responsibility upon the volunteers.

Both Confederate and Union newspapers expressed solidarity with the surgeons, more accurately representing surgeons' frustrations than the soldiers' frightening experiences within the Medical Departments. The *Christian Recorder*, for instance, confirmed the "great difficulty in obtaining medicines" and the "loud and deep . . . mutterings of some of the surgeons against the red-tape system which prevails among the medical officials." Such reporting reiterated the complaints of many surgeons that circumstances, not incompetence, prevented them from doing their jobs. The job of surgeon was portrayed as taxing, complex, and admirable: "In a word, anything relating to the health, diet, clothing, cleanliness, and comfort of the sick, devolves upon the surgeon and his assistants."[136] The *Daily Dispatch* also had praise for surgeons, deeming them "a very ill-used set of people. They are abused when men are well, sent for when they are sick, and rarely receive what they deserve." Further, just as surgeons and commanders tended to emphasize care for the wounded over the sick, the papers touted the "Surgeon at Work" on the battlefield as most distinguished. "Of all officers the surgeon is often the one who requires most nerve and most courage," proclaimed *Harper's Weekly*.[137] Hospitals were likewise shown in a positive light. They were "on the whole, much more comfortable than could be supposed possible, where woman's presence and invaluable services are, with few exceptions, not to be found."[138]

Even when presented with a clear opportunity to critique the quality of surgeons, reporters tended to err on the side of supporting them. The *Valley Spirit*, for instance, portrayed Union medical reforms as misguided in seeking to enlist the most qualified physicians. One May article explained that a Harrisburg-based medical board had attempted to examine candidates for military surgeon positions. Though local doctors signed up, they subsequently refused to sit for the exam, because they could not remember the more trivial information from medical school. The article claimed that those who could most easily pass the exams were, in fact, medical students rather than distinguished physicians with practical experience.[139] The article thus professed support for the old model of professional physicians, in which reputation and experience mattered more than scientific knowledge. But for common soldiers, this was another reminder that the middle to upper classes closed ranks over who administered proper health care.

Overall, the official medical systems were bewilderingly complex and guarded by the cultural values of those who had power over common soldiers. It was therefore difficult for soldiers to navigate the labyrinthine bureaucracy and advocate for their best care. In the void of health protection that resulted, soldiers were confronted with a dire choice: accept responsibility for their own bodies or succumb to illness and possibly death. Longing for the personal nature of prewar family care, many soldiers would attempt to create an informal network of medical knowledge and health care that was responsive to the new environment of war.

4

Becoming a Seasoned Soldier

Given the tremendous environmental pressures on mental and physical health and the unreliable nature of the Confederate and Union military medical systems, common soldiers attempted to reconstruct personal, informal networks of environmental information and health care based on their prewar experiences. This unofficial system would be based on spontaneous opportunity, experiential knowledge, and the aid of fellow soldiers and individuals near the front and at home. While it was often impossible for most soldiers, except Virginians stationed near their homes or those on furlough, to receive physical nursing from their loved ones, correspondence served as a proxy for family care, while comrades or individuals traveling with the armies or residing nearby could offer personal advice and attention. The difference between those who made up the unofficial network of self-care and those who composed the Medical Departments was that the former were generally not entangled in bureaucracy or military goals; rather, they were focused on helping the soldier to survive. Because of individualized support and because of the self-care emphasis on prevention, the fully seasoned soldier had the best chance of remaining healthy and whole in 1862 Virginia.

Of the healthiest and happiest soldiers in this study, a number of trends are apparent. Most important: the healthiest men practiced a wide range of self-care techniques, and equal numbers were Confederate and Union soldiers. Further, those who remained physically healthy were also mentally healthy.[1] Men in blue and gray proved remarkably resourceful in their habits and developed the same sorts of techniques. Some habits were simply extensions of civilian life, while others required a cultural shift to master. Sometimes self-care became a group experience, even inciting competition and pride, while other practices were conducted alone, secretly, or in pairs. Self-care could both prevent and treat illness. Some techniques abounded on the march, while others were only useful when in camp. It is not entirely clear why some men adopted effective self-care routines, while others passively accepted their fates. The evidence suggests that certain circumstances of service proved more conducive to practicing self-care, such as the flexibility of a cavalryman or officer. Officer oversight or the availability of people to participate in the informal network of care played a major role. No doubt, personal resilience and genetic factors also influenced the decision to practice self-care and one's overall susceptibility to disease and melancholy. Finally, the fact remains that some humans respond to hardship with resignation, while others respond with resilience, lending some credence to the contemporary idea that a positive attitude could bolster health.

This is not to say that self-care was a panacea. There were a few cases in which soldiers practiced extensive and varied self-care routines but could not ward off illness and debilitating sadness. Variables such as age, health before enlistment, and the precise locations to which one's regiment was deployed played a role in the outcome of self-care. Also, it is important to bear in mind that the numbers of sick soldiers far exceeded the numbers of healthy soldiers despite widespread use of certain self-care techniques. Therefore, self-care was only so effective in mitigating the environment of war. For instance, if a person bathed regularly but did not drain his camp of moisture to prevent mosquito infestations, then even if he avoided diarrhea he was still likely to contract malaria. Self-care did, however, provide a means of actively pursuing environmental seasoning on the way to becoming a veteran, a badge of honor for Civil War soldiers.

EXPERIMENTING WITH SELF-CARE

Confederate Pvt. Randolph McKim was encamped with the Army of Northern Virginia in April of 1862. Miserable, wet, and cold, he did a surprising thing—he broke through some ice by a railroad and plunged his body into the freezing depths below. "Bathing was a rare privilege," he remarked, a habit worth such a sacrifice. Why he would willingly entice hypothermia was subsequently revealed in his account. "Under the genial sun we would soon forget our miseries and enjoy the beautiful scenery sometimes spread out before us." Prior to this incident, the men had been "almost broken down with the weather" of that "unfriendly spring."[2] Bathing, therefore, provided important psychological benefits to the weary soldier. Likewise did 13th Massachusetts infantryman Pvt.

Ephraim A. Wood's Valley diary read as downright cheery compared to the average journal. Refreshed from bathing every two to four days, Wood regarded blazing ninety-degree temperatures as merely "warm."[3]

While some self-care techniques would require a cultural shift to execute, bathing was generally an extension of civilian life, though perhaps slightly more common among the middle to upper classes.[4] Yet under the circumstances of war, the stakes of a bath were substantially raised and the ability to wash was hampered by the regimentation of army life. For those on the march, orders to bathe were issued with dangerous infrequence — sometimes weeks apart — if one did not slip out of the ranks. Skipping a bath meant, for instance, a higher chance of succumbing to sunstroke. Sunstroke, an affliction far underestimated in the *U.S. Medical and Surgical History of the War*, could be deadly, and, at the very least, caused soldiers to drop to the wayside unable to perform their duties.[5]

A Pennsylvanian on the Peninsula, Lt. Jacob W. Haas went down into a ravine and sat with his feet in the water when the heat became so unbearable that "several of the men became sun-blinded."[6] Subsequently, he was able to carry on, while his comrades had to abandon the ranks. Pvt. Edmund DeWitt Patterson of the 9th Alabama, who could not stop for a full bath, applied the same principle with the water he had on hand: "On the march I became so overheated that I could scarcely catch my breath, and I felt that I would faint, but happily I had a canteen of water and stretching myself on my back in the shade of a tree, I unbuttoned my shirt and poured the canteen of water in my bossom, which soon relieved me."[7] While the men did not necessarily refer to bathing as good sanitation but rather as a means to increase comfort, in reality bathing critically prevented the spread of bacteria and helped to detach the insects responsible for conveying disease. Sanitary Commission inspector Samuel G. Howe noted that at least Union soldiers were rationed soap, though its quality was "wretchedly bad."[8] With or without soap, the benefits of washing were manifest. One Marylander, Cpl. Washington Hands, believed his bath helped revive him after suffering the "excruciating agony" of camp fever. "The first day that I was able to go about, I hunted up a stream of water and took a good bath and made a change of under clothes."[9] Refreshed, Hands was able to return to soldiering. Some men who refused to bathe were coerced by their officers. Sgt. William H. West of the 6th Maine Infantry explained that "Frank Campbell was detailed to clean J. A. Longfellow. He took him to the brook and made him wash and left his clothes there."[10] One reason some soldiers were reluctant to bathe was their resistance to forfeiting privacy, as bathing was often a public event.

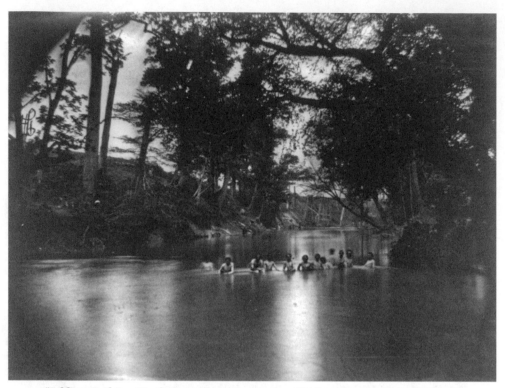

"Soldiers Bathing, North Anna River, Va.—Ruins of Railroad Bridge in Background,"
May 1864 (No. B815-763, Civil War Collection, Library of Congress)

As these stories suggest, those who located water for bathing were also more inclined to wash their clothes, further improving hygiene. Uniforms provided critical protection from the elements, and it was vital to maintain them. Doing one's laundry, however, was one of the more difficult self-care tactics for the men to master, not because it required exceptional skill, but because it compelled a shift in gender norms. Before the war, laundry was considered women's work, and indeed, many units continued to have access to a company washer; however, soldiers often had to pay up to fifty cents a month for their services.[11] The savvy soldier realized that opportunities to wash were rare and water sources scarce. Fifth Virginian Pvt. Thomas M. Smiley wrote in his July diary in his entry on the twenty-fifth that the "men are now all out washing thier clothes it being the first oportunity for six weeks."[12] Some proved more reluctant to make such a transition in expectations. After eleven full months of service, 17th Virginian Pvt. William Smith, who had long benefited from being stationed near home, finally acquiesced and did his own washing. He lamented, "We now begin to realize the unpleasantness of being cut off from all communication with home."[13]

It was not only Virginians who adapted with reluctance, knowing that their families were often just a short journey away. Pennsylvanian cavalryman Pvt. Allen L. Bevan made the typical rookie mistake of casting off his clothes in a forced march. Then, stuck with a filthy and flimsy set, he hoped to get his clothes washed for him, believing clean clothes would make him feel "all right again." Instead he finally bought new clothes, and yet his problem of keeping them clean did not vanish. "I did not lose my new flannel shirt but have some trouble now for to get them washed and I had to wash two the other day myself." His reluctance at last gave way to pride: "Bully for me," he wrote, exuberantly pleased with his own progress as a soldier.[14] Pvt. William Stilwell, a Georgian, was likewise enamored of his newfound laundry skills when he wrote to his wife: "Molly, you would have been surprised to have seen me and Bob McDonald washing out shorts and drawers the other day. We did not have any clothes but what we had on for eight or ten days and we went about half mile from camp, pulled off stark naked and went out to wash like good fellows, dried and put them on again. We are very good hands at the business."[15] The price of failing to achieve this adaptation was grave: "I have not slept with my pants off for above 2 months to which I attribute an itching & burning of the flesh," Lieutenant Haydon bemoaned, probably suffering from a case of scabies.[16] Pvt. John D. Billings's memoir, often keen in its analysis, captured the cultural shift best: "It may be asked what kind of a figure the men cut as washerwomen. Well some of them were awkward . . . but necessity is a capital teacher."[17]

Uniforms indeed provided a frontline of defense against pests and exposure, but they required more upkeep than simple washing. Pennsylvanian Pvt. Thomas Langstroth explained, "The sun comes down to us poor mortals with more force than I ever felt before. it is hot enough to day to cook eggs in its power, my head suffers sorely with the heat." He believed a new set of clothes would ease his suffering. "If I had some thin clothes with me I should be more comfortable but it would be very uncertain to reach me so they had better not be sent. The most clothes in the carpet bag got wet with salt water and are spoilt as I did not find it out till they were all mouldy musty and partly roten."[18] If Langstroth dreamed of clean, weather-appropriate attire, he was not alone. Many soldiers purchased new uniforms in towns on their meager pay, or, as Langstroth was tempted, requested clothes from home. Clothes could be spoils of war from a vanquished foe, though Virginia artillerist Pvt. James P. Williams eschewed such "plundering." "Some of the fellows filled their knapsacks with nice clean Yankee clothes but I had no desire myself to wear their clothes."[19] Still, other soldiers took pride in their newfound abilities to mend their tattered clothing, which had once again been women's work before the war. At one point Private McClellan of Alabama claimed he would never need a wife, considering his newfound domestic skills: "I have learned to do my own cooking and sewing and I can make up my own bed," he boasted.[20] He changed his mind, however, shortly thereafter, when he admitted that even a man of his considerable talents still became lonely.

Perhaps the most storied item in one's arsenal of clothing was shoes, and the men who attended to their feet bolstered their own health significantly. While improper shoes could lead to severe discomfort and plunging morale on the march, a lack of shoes could also expose a soldier to hookworm, which enter the body through bare feet. Both Union and Confederate soldiers complained of the symptoms: rashes, shortness of breath, cough, gastrointestinal distress, anemia, and protein loss—the latter two of which might also contribute to lackluster spirits. Pvt. Alvin N. Brackett of the 1st Maine cavalry was so tired of tramping around Front Royal in the rain without dry clothes that he requested from home "a pare of rubber boots that would come up to my ass."[21] An action as seemingly trivial as drying one's feet could make a measurable difference in a soldier's well-being. Musician Lewis C. Shepard of the 7th Massachusetts remarked in his diary, "I noticed I feel pretty tired. My feet are just as wet as they can be." Shepard changed his stockings and put on his "Government slippers." He immediately felt better and remarked with satisfaction upon how his comrades looked far more bedraggled than he.[22]

While bathing and laundry were sometimes conducted in pairs or groups, bed and tent construction were almost always the products of mass camaraderie. Arranging the perfect sleeping accommodations ignited competitiveness and individuality and garnered great pride among Civil War soldiers. Some of the more creative beds, usually designed to keep out moisture, involved an imaginative array of issued goods and natural surroundings. In a postscript, Massachusetts infantryman Private Blackington explained to his sister, Hannah, how real soldiers slept: "I must make my bed (put a handful of leaves down on the ground in our tent and throw a rubber blanket on top of them and cover ourselves with the woolen blanket and sleep as sound as we would in the softest bed)."[23] Pvt. Charles Perkins of the 1st Massachusetts used a configuration so complex to mitigate his rheumatism that it encumbers the imagination. "Bed as follows My rubber blanket laid on ground Blouse Dress coat & overcoat in cape over my head Rolled in Woolen blanket & Whit's Rubber over Both of us Both ends of tent open & me laid across it."[24] Private McClellan hoped to cure his cold caught from "sleeping upon the ground" with a better bunk design made of driving forks in the ground and laying poles and wooden planks across them.[25] What the soldiers did not fully comprehend is that the techniques not only prevented them from becoming saturated by rain in one's sleep, but also kept one's body off camp soil, which often harbored parasites and bacteria, especially when rain had contaminated the dirt with latrine waste. Lt. Campbell Brown and his sleeping companion had one of the more bizarre remedies for drenched bedclothes. When a "fearfully hard rain came up," Brown recorded that "the India-rubber blanket, under which we were sleeping in a skirt of woods not far from the depot, became so full of water in the hollow made by its sinking down between us, that I woke thinking Turner was pulling the cover off me." Because the two men had already become so accustomed to soldier life, "the rain had not fairly waked us, our heads being covered, and we were much surprised to find a gallon or more of water in the blanket. Both of us drank out of it, & then emptied it & went to sleep."[26] If they could not beat the rain, they used it—to satisfy their thirsts. They had truly become seasoned soldiers, able to make one man's problem another's solution.

When it came to tents, often men relied upon each other to button together half shelters into more suitable coverage. They also improvised with surrounding foliage to construct entrances, roofs, and chimneys and were sometimes surprised by how quickly an encampment could deforest a particular area.[27] While Confederates were more chronically deprived of tents, both Federals and Confederates occasionally had to make do without shelter (as far too many soldiers abandoned tents on the march because of their weight). These men improvised accordingly. Capt. Edward Rush Young of the 1st Virginia Artillery and his men "spread our blankets upon the ground reserving a few to cover up our heads & shelter us from the impending storm. . . . The clouds gathered in blackness above our heads & poured out their vials of wrath in the form of electricity & rain upon our devoted heads. We covered up our head & ears in our blankets & hudling together tried to keep as dry & comfortable as possible."[28] This protection was not half as effective as taking shelter under a tree, whether to protect from rain or heat or sometimes even the stench of battle. Private Perkins found that when the decay of dead horses overpowered his camp, he sought out a swamp magnolia, which pleasantly perfumed his slumber.[29]

Captain Young's experience of sleeping out in the rain with his men calls to attention an important point about self-care: officers (including surgeons) also practiced self-care techniques but with slightly lower stakes, as they enjoyed critical advantages over their men. Initially, officers and field hospitals were issued wall tents, which had four upright sides, but these were often discarded as inconvenient for travel.[30] Maj. Frank B. Jones of the 2nd Virginia suffered from poor health but could seek out comfort when he needed it most. When it was rainy in March and "very disagreeable," he had the option to go "into a log church," where he "slept very comfortably." So hearty was he from his rest that he proclaimed the church "a romantic spot," a sign of improved spirits. An enlisted man in his situation would have been accused of straggling and potentially punished. When he had another hard day of it in April—"Sun was hot. Felt depressed and miserable. Had suffered the day before from a violent nervous headache"—he was "fortunate enough to get into a carpenter shop and [sleep] comfortably on the dry floor," while the "men bivouacked on the wet ground." He realized that his men had no such safety valve, at least without considerable disciplinary risk. For instance, when rain plagued his regiment that same month, he wrote, "Am much pleased with Peytunia, [his horse] she is a fine animal and carried me today through the mud and swollen streams notably. This is the 4th day of rain. How do men stand such exposure!"[31] In addition to the fact that officers slept far more often in buildings and traveled on horseback, they also enjoyed superior rations and received more prompt and complete care from surgeons. Surgeons themselves acknowledged their advantage over the rank and file. Surgeon Castleman wrote, "To-night, after a march of twelve miles through mud and rain, the men lie out without shelter, except the little tents debris, which in time of rain are good for nothing." He shuddered "when I think of them, exposed, after a hard day's march, to the driving storm. And whilst they are thus exposed, I feel almost guilty that I am in a fine hotel, by a fine coal fire, 'comfortable and cozy.'"[32]

Winter presented a particular challenge for common soldiers to achieve proper protection from the elements and, therefore, inspired the most elaborate sleeping quarters. A soldier reported to the *Boston Journal* how Union winter camps were arranged: "Boys would chum together, usually four, sometimes two, but not often six. They would go into the woods and cut down some good-sized young trees."[33] In January 1862, an artist for *Harper's Weekly* similarly depicted soldiers working in teams to haul wood and construct log huts, the pouring rain failing to dissuade them from their cheerful teamwork.[34] Once the men had acquired the building materials, the trees "were cut into logs, each of which was neatly cleft in two. Then these logs were notched at the ends and placed upon another,

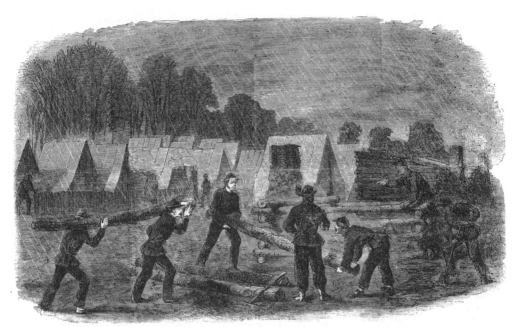

"Building Huts for the Army of the Potomac" (Harper's Weekly, January 18, 1862)

with the smooth side in, and the rounded, bark-covered portion out." No log cabin was complete without a fireplace: "The big cob chimney was the poetical feature. It was built of short sticks, laid criss cross, 'cob' fashion, and to finish it, for a cap-piece, a barrel was stuck on top."[35] Though Pvt. Robert T. Hubard and his 3rd Virginian comrades lacked log cabins, they did possess "good tents and owing to easy transportation and plenty of sawmills we had plank furnished to us to make bed-steads and floors. We learned then the art of making various sorts of wooden chimneys, and these kept the tents quite dry." A competition to develop the most effective chimney arose. "The most popular mode was to build them up three sides to the arch, then run a four-corner stem; and, driving stobs in the ground inside about eight inches from the sides of the chimney, place the dirt into the space between, very tightly. The stem we afterwards daubed. The fire would soon burn the stobs away and leave a wall of firmly cemented dirt to protect the wooden frame."[36]

Not only did soldiers attempt to protect their bodies from the elements, but they also carefully observed the environs of camp, harnessing resources and intervening to improve their circumstances. For instance, a soldier near Yorktown expressed gratitude for his fine location. "We still remain in camp, and are comfortable, that is for soldiers, as circumstances will admit. Our tents are of good material and keep out the rain, and the camp is situation on rather high ground, therefore the water runs off." What was even better about this camp was the water: "a small stream . . . supplied by pure springs, from which we get plenty of water for drinking and cooking purposes," and "a thick wood of pine, with their ever-green foliage; elm-trees, which were soon robbed of their bark to satisfy the chewing propensities of the men; sassafras bushes, the roots of which are pleasant to eat, and are therefore pulled up without regard to quantity." While the camp was pleasant for this regiment, for the next troops there would be little left—" The wood is now getting thinner every day, falling a sacrifice to our axes, and used by the cooks to keep up their fires, and by us as a means to warm ourselves when it is necessary."[37] Twelfth Massachusetts infantryman Cpl. Joseph E. Blake noted that his was "a most butifull place," a "good Camp Ground," owing to fresh water, berries, shade, and a lack of malarial winds.[38] Many soldiers agreed with the popular medical opinion that changing one's locale to higher and more salubrious ground would improve faltering health and plummeting spirits. For example, Lieutenant Haydon noted, "We are moving our camp. . . . A clear puddle here will turn black & be covered with green scum within 10 hours after it falls."[39] Thus, men analyzed the health of the camp assigned them and efficiently extracted resources.

But when soldiers found themselves in insalubrious camps that they could not evacuate, some men directly intervened to alter their environments. Pvt. David Watson from Virginia explained to his mother, "During some of the few good days we have had I have had our camp tolerably drained and hauled up a good deal of sand from the beach and spread it in front of the quarters so that walking about is not quite so bad as it was at first when you stepped out of doors into a mud hole whenever you went out." If the private could not relocate, he would bring the higher ground to him. Watson and others like him did not realize it, but draining a camp was one of the most effective ways to reduce malaria-carrying mosquitoes. He did note, "I think we have all kept remarkably well for people wading in water and necessarily a great deal exposed as most of the men are."[40] Private Fletcher from Texas similarly remembered that his unit laid cordwood down, as outdoor flooring, to prevent the moisture of the Chickahominy swamps from seeping into camp.[41] These men both reaped the benefits of being in camp rather than on the march. Directly managing one's environment took time and effort, and the transient bivouacs of marches often did not provide the opportunity for either.

In addition to altering their environments, soldiers also gained some amount of control over their surroundings—both in camp and on the march—simply by educating themselves about the local flora, avoiding what was potentially harmful and even selecting medicinal herbs. For a Pennsylvanian such as Aaron Bachman, identifying poisonous plants was an acquired skill. "I suffered from a severe case of ivy poison," he remembered. "I had slept in a fence corner that was full of the poison, and had to have a doctor's care to get me over it. After that I watched the fence corners before sleeping in them."[42] Other soldiers sought out plants with medicinal value that they perhaps recognized from back home or the domestic manuals. Pvt. Lorenzo N. Pratt, of the 1st New York Light Artillery, explained to his father that when sick in the New Market area, he "got hold of some of that spice root and sasafraz root and I chawed it and it made me well."[43] Based on Pratt's attention to the crops of the "secesh" farms he came across, his knowledge of the roots was likely gleaned in his rural farming days in New York, as it is indigenous across eastern North America. It is difficult to identify Pratt's illness, but sassafras can indeed be medicinally used to treat pain and rheumatism. His relief may well have been genuine.

In addition to learning about flora, soldiers quickly became experts on how to eradicate insects, be they flies, mosquitoes, ticks, lice, or chiggers. Though they were not yet aware of the price of certain insect bites for human health, they were all too cognizant of the incredible discomfort and annoyance bugs engendered. It is telling that years later when many soldiers sat down to write their recollections about 1862, one of their most vivid memories of camp life was exterminating pests. Private Bellard recalled "when an army of Virginia mosquitoes made a general attack on our post, that was on the edge of the wood." First the soldiers took up a kind of wild group dance to scare them off: "We were completely surrounded and had to keep our arms continually in motion trying to brush them off." This failing, they "built a wood fire, making plenty of smoke in the hopes of smoking them out, but it was no go, as they would bite us even after we got into the smoke." Resigned, the men "wrapped ourselves up in our blankets, leaving nothing but our eyes and nose exposes and stood it best as we could until daylight, when they retreated. They were the largest specimens I ever saw and the most blood thirsty as well."[44] In such situations, there was something to be said for solidarity. Even if the men only achieved limited success at staving off their afflicters, they, at least, concocted a reasonable string of distractions from focusing on the bites they received. Of course, if they succeeded in routing the mosquitoes, they then lowered their chances of contracting malaria.[45]

Flies were par for the course in a war replete with dead and wounded bodies, mobile latrines, and animal offal, but they were also dangerous, as they transported typhoid fever and intestinal diseases on their tiny feet. Following the battles of the Seven Days, Private Fletcher remembered how the aftermath of fighting could precipitate a rush of flies on the march. As the men were "passing over and near the battlefield, seeing the destruction that it brought to man, beast and property," they suffered from "the awful stench that at times would great one's nostrils, and in this instance myriads of flies." When they camped a few miles from Richmond, they were no longer "affected with the odor," but the insects remained. These were not your everyday flies. "They were something less than the common housefly, and when they bit or sucked it left a stinging sensation, and when one lay down for a nap in daytime he was forced to cover up, as it were, head and ears."[46] Flies are attracted to mucous membranes, and covering up the face did help to dissuade them from launching their attacks on the sleeping soldiers.

Private Fletcher also had an unsavory experience with lice, which led to his fervent attempt to eradicate them. "The picket line was a short distance to the front," he remembered, "and from all appearances the place had been occupied by troops for some time, and by some who were very lousy; for lice could be seen crawling on the grass leaves and body of the trees." He noted a sad vulnerability in his self-care regime: "Here I learned that in moving and occupying the same grounds occupied by others, that cleanliness was no bar to lice." But as consolation "the color of the Confederate uniform had the advantage over the Federal in not showing them when on the outside of the clothing." While the Texans may have concealed their newfound lousy-ness in their uniforms, the fact was they were beginning to itch. "Our plan was, when they got so thick that they were hardly bearable, to make a fire . . . and hold the garment over the blaze and from the heat they would drop off, be burned, or be ready for the next fellow. If one was well stocked with big fat fellows, it would remind him of popping corn."[47] While the remedy was only partially effective with lice, the fire had a secondary benefit; the U.S. Sanitary Commission recommended building campfires "for preventing annoyance from insects," because some insects were dissuaded by the smoke.[48]

Private Billings similarly described soldiers' attempts to rid themselves of lice with a kind of progressive group effort. "After the first discovery, the . . . soldier would appoint himself an investigating committee of one to sit with closed door. . . . There he would seat himself taking his garments across his knees in turn, conscientiously doing his (k)nitting work, inspecting every fibre with the scrutiny of a dealer in broadcloths." In the winter months, Billings claimed the "skirmishing" would happen indoors but in warm weather, "the woods usually found near camps full of [the men] sprinkled about singly or in social parties of two or three slaying their victims by the thousands." When picking off the pests didn't work, Billings said the men resolved to procure a new uniform and burn the old one, hanging on a bush. He also explained the merits and drawbacks of boiling water, which was said to "cook the millions yet unborn." Men claimed they still saw the critters "creeping on garments taken out of boiling water," and that the only remedy was to add salt to accomplish "their destruction."[49] Other men simply made removing unwanted insects a part of their morning routine. A soldier from the 11th Massachusetts wrote home on May 20, 1862, from the Peninsula about how he began a typical day. "Here in the morning when I get up, I begin the day by taking off my clothes and picking out the wood ticks & ground—well-say insects, and then . . . I am ready for a wash and breakfast."[50]

Many of the remaining self-care techniques ultimately revolved around controlling what one put in one's body—crucial to avoiding all manner of disease, from diarrhea and dysentery to typhoid fever to scurvy. "Whiskey is for drinking, water is for fighting over," it is alleged Mark Twain said, and this could certainly be applied to the soldiers in 1862 Virginia. Finding drinkable water (or sometimes any water at all) was a tremendous challenge, yet clean water prevented the most common and deadly of diseases and, of course, dehydration. Soldiers were not fully aware of the price of drinking foul water, but they did detest it. Pvt. Kinchen Jahu Carpenter wrote, "It is impossible for me to describe what our troops have gone through. Hunger, thirst and fatigue was awful. We would drink water from a stream that had dead horses in it. When you are so very thirsty, any kind of water is good."[51] They feared water that tasted and smelled rank and were equally suspicious of what one soldier called "change of water," which could lead to disease much like change of climate.[52]

Soldiers thus devised creative solutions to problems with their water supply. Pvt. Oliver Norton was confronted with "roily swamp water," so he cleverly boiled it into coffee.[53] Lt. Tully McCrea had another remedy for bad camp water—buying it. To his dear Belle he wrote, "At first we drank spring water, but it had such a nauseating taste that I scarcely drank it. After this we bought our water from a volunteer regiment that had dug a well."[54] When Corporal Blake and his comrades discovered pure water at Warrenton, their morale notably improved: "It is a most butifull place here, their is plenty of good watter here and a soldier thinks more of good water than any thing else."[55] Those who could not discover suitable water made their own luck. Lieutenant Haydon explained, "We now have three good wells which supply an abundance of excellent water adding greatly to our health & comfort."[56] Digging wells, however, was a luxury reserved for encampments of longer duration. Sgt. David C. Ashley, a cavalryman on the Peninsula, might have found himself at a disadvantage having to share water with the horses of his unit, but he made up for the lack of water by stealing milk from local farms.[57]

Other soldiers soon discovered the other half of the Twain proverb—whiskey—as a replacement for fetid water; the uses of whiskey went beyond satisfying thirst, however. Whiskey was considered medicinal and even prescribed by doctors and rationed by commanders. While the alcohol had some ability to kill bacteria, its benefits as a centuries-old battlefield panacea had more to do with pain relief. Pvt. David Bell of the 105th Pennsylvania Infantry wrote in a letter that "we drew to rations of whiskey each day by order of Gen. McClelland," to help mitigate the ill effects of exposure.[58] Another Pennsylvanian private explained, "Once when I felt most like giving it up, Dr. Livingston called me out of the ranks and administered a good dose of whiskey. It completely revived me for a time."[59] Among self-medicators was Maj. Frank B. Jones, for whom a dose of whiskey gave him the strength to go on. "Felt very badly all day, but with a flask of whiskey wich W. S. J. had given me I was enabled to ride and attend to duty."[60] As Jones's case reveals, officers had readier access to whiskey, again providing them with privileges that enlisted men lacked. And yet, as discussed earlier, alcohol use could quickly lead down a slippery slope to ineffective soldiering. It was an example of self-care, or at least self-administered medicine, that could improve the way a man felt temporarily but with few long-term benefits.

One of the most important self-care techniques in 1862 was foraging for fruits and vegetables, since the early rations did not provide adequate vitamin C. After three to eight months of insufficient diet, armies could become plagued with weakened, sore, and dispirited soldiers—men suffering from scurvy. Some were aware of the benefits of fruits and vegetables as anti-scourbotics, while others simply indulged a hankering for berries, peaches, apples, and lemons. The Valley's abundance of fruit made it easier for soldiers to improve their diets, but soldiers on the Peninsula also proved resourceful in supplementing their rations. Sergeant Ashley enjoyed the strawberries growing in Yorktown on May 31, and Pvt. Jacob Blackington was blessed by the ingenuity of a messmate.[61] "Jake is out picking green swamp berries to stew. We have plenty of them here and

Jake and me have stewed berries every day for a week or more," he wrote to his sister. Blackington proved that he kept his eye on potential forage, explaining, "Cherries are beginning to color and will be ripe in 10 days or so."[62] Cpl. John H. Bevan explained that camping was more conducive to foraging than marching. Our "style of living has changed considerably since we came into camp; while on the march we got no soft bread at all it being hard bread or crackers." Now, the men relished the presence of dewberries "in great abundance, whole fields which have not been farmed for a few years are full of them. We can now go out and pick a couple of quarts in about a half hour or so, and we have been living here more than a week and eating dewberries nearly every day."[63] His spirits noticeably improved.

The fact that scurvy had both mental and generalized physical consequences made it an elusive and confusing disease to soldiers (not to mention to physicians). For instance, Pvt. Charles Perkins was puzzled about what exactly ailed him. Vegetables seemed to spell instant if temporary relief: "Monday Aug 4 took Dose of opium Never had the Di so bad before [at] Dinner . . . relished the vegetables very much." When his throat became sore the next day, he continued to rely upon vegetables and fruits for reprieve, purchasing some apples, onions, plums, and lemons.[64] Most likely, Perkins avoided scurvy but suffered from another ailment, as he was sick nearly his entire stay on the Peninsula. Capt. Oliver Wendell Holmes was ordered to consume lemons by a doctor, but he would soon learn to practice the habit on his own. To his mother he wrote, "In my own case the scorbutic symptoms are not in general specific so much as they are traceable to the same cause (want of fresh food). . . . It's rather funny to drink lemonade for disorder of the bowels though! As the doctors order. The homesickness wh. I mentioned in my last they say is one of the first symptoms of scurvy."[65] In these cases, soldiers learned by trial and error, basing their self-care regimes on experience and advice passed among the ranks.

SOLDIERS AS NURSES

In addition to devising techniques to prevent and treat sickness and demoralization, self-care involved the construction of informal networks of care. It has already been made evident that soldiers learned from one another, but they also preferred comrades when illness struck. Some soldiers did know their regimental surgeon from home and considered these men to be more friend than doctor. But many men opted to be nursed by a comrade, reminiscent of home care, as an alternative to the regimental or general hospital. Soldiers were well aware of each other's ailments—not to mention those who were feigning illness—and proved attentive to those in need. Confederate cavalryman Pvt. John Gill revealed how soldiers' first thoughts in sickness were to be nursed in a clean bed by someone who cared personally for their well-being: "I think it was in the early part of September that I was stricken down with typhoid fever. I was ill for more than nine weeks. Most of the time I lay on the hard ground, receiving very little attention from anybody. My life was almost despaired of." When he approached the surgeon and asked "what were my chances of recovery . . . his reply was not cheerful. I said to him, 'Doctor, if you will only take me to a house, strip me of these vile clothes filled with vermin and put me in a clean bed, I shall live.'" A "providential" twist led to a local gentleman offering to take some of the 1st Maryland's sick into his house, where Gill recovered.[66]

While good fortune spared Gill, most soldiers had to make their own luck by depending upon their comrades. Sergeant Pryor happened to like his surgeon a good deal: "Dr. Beveridge gave me phisic & attended to me right. He is a good doctor & a nice man and I have reason to believe he is a good friend of mine," but he recognized that his lieutenant was more instrumental in his recovery from illness. "Dawson is a true friend. As soon as Capt. Hawkins left he asked me to come up & sleep with him while I was sick. He fed me from his table any thing he could get. Il stick to him, for I know that heel befriend me." Pryor knew he was lucky: "There is so many of my friends of the com. died & been discharge and are absent at the different hospitals. There is now in camp 49 of our company."[67] In Pryor's case, he was able to benefit from tapping into the resources of a commissioned officer. The best officers did take a personal interest in the health of their men. Capt. Josiah C. Fuller of the 32nd Massachusetts wrote of nursing his men as though it were simply one of his duties. After he was evidently thanked by those at home for looking after Pvt. Robert H. Barnes from his regiment, he responded, "You write me R. Barnes wrote home concerning me. He was a little sick . . . when he wrote and thought others did not attend to him as [well as I]. I am pleased to have people think well of me but would not be pleased much less elated by flattery. I mean to look after my men and all others as far as I can."[68] Fuller and many other regimental officers knew their soldiers' families from home and were well aware that neglecting even one man could result in a thorough chastising via correspondence.

The relationship between officers and their subordinates in times of need went both ways. Some officers found that their men rewarded compassionate leadership by nursing superiors back to health. Non-commissioned officer Corporal Hands explained, "I was 2nd Corporal in charge of a squad or mess, and an old Scotch man by the name of [Mac?] . . . nursed me like a father. I had to report every morning to Hospital call and be prescribed the medicine . . . mostly of Blue mass. . . . [Mac?] fed me an [?] black coffee which gradually brought me through in [conjunction?] with his good nursing and attention."[69] Hands may have been treated by his surgeon, but it was the private who brought him through his illness. Similarly, Capt. James A. Sheeran suffered cruelly from pneumonia along with many other Confederate soldiers, who died at the time from the disease. "Fortunately for myself, by solicitation and consent, I secured a good and attentive nurse from my company, in the person of Addison Lanford, who was my messmate. Doubtless without such attention as he gave me, I would have shared the same fate of others who needed better attention."[70] Interesting in his description is that he actually requested the aid, as one might request a doctor's care. Though Sheeran could have solicited a surgeon's care, he preferred his comrade's. In such a way was sickness a class leveler.[71] Though privates may have been more vulnerable to falling ill, when it came to receiving care soldiers relied on the man who was most willing and able to provide assistance regardless of rank.

Privates commonly cared for each other, as they were bunkmates and knew firsthand how dreadful exposure could lead to disease. The sickly Pvt. Charles Perkins relied on his messmate, "Holden," to exchange rations so that Perkins could have something he could stomach despite his persistent diarrhea. "Bowels trouble me again owing to water. Am not very strong. Supper of crackers and water. Holden gave me a few crackers very good."[72] In July on the Peninsula, Georgian Pvt. Stilwell was ill and wrote, "The boys are very kind to me. We have nothing but tent flies to keep us dry. The boys hang up blankets to keep the rain off me." In August, stationed near Richmond, he was still sick "with bilious fever and measles." He explained that "it is a bad thing to be sick in camp but I have fared as well as could be expected in camps. Bob sent off and bought straw for me to lie on and hung up blankets to keep the rain off." Following the incident, he praised Bob as "a good friend of mine."[73] Some of the enlistees, such as the Bevans of the 1st Pennsylvania Reserve Calvary, joined the same regiments as their family members and felt an added responsibility to tend to one another. When John wrote home on February 2, 1862, it was clear that his mother had inquired after his care of his brother. John responded, "You advise me to take care of Al's health and also of my own; this I always do as far as I can."[74]

Not every soldier was sympathetic toward their sick comrades. If a man complained too much, fellow soldiers might suspect him of malingering.[75]

Pvt. Simon B. Hulbert of the 100th New York Infantry wrote home that "Ett wants to know how old Winters is. Well now, since he had the measles he is about poor. He is clear discouraged, does not move unless he is drove, & he is telling all the time how bad he feels. I almost get out of patience with him sometimes because he is so much of the time in my way & I hope he will get in better spirits before long. I do not know but he will Die before long. He is getting poor as a shad & he makes a face most all the time, just as Aunt Sarah Brown used too [*sic*]. I do not know but he is sick, but if he would stir I think he would enjoy better heath & then he swears so much."[76] Apparently "Old Winters" was not doing his part to become seasoned. Rather than receiving sympathy, he was shunned by comrades. Interestingly, Reverend Stewart commented in hindsight, "The inexperienced may be ready to suppose that, from their mutually exposed condition, soldiers would be very sympathetic, and disposed readily to assist and comfort each other. To the very opposite of this, there seems, however, a strong tendency. The soldier seldom acts toward the sick, the dying and the dead, as he was wont to do at home."[77] As it was simply untrue that soldiers "seldom" cared for each other, Stewart may have been remembering soldiers' impatience with malingerers, or he may have been recasting himself in a more heroic role that emphasized his middle-class superiority in the realm of suffering.

In many cases, the men helped transport their sick friends or family members in the ranks to a hospital or civilian home to make sure they received proper care. They also delivered to them food and supplies when away from the ranks. Occasionally, these men were granted leave to accompany or visit the sick, and other times they were not but left the ranks in any case. Private Davis from Minnesota wrote to his sister about his careful attendance to a friend. "I went over to Isaac to day and found him in the hospital. The doctor says he has a slow fever, and is not dangerous. He has fallen away very much. I try to get him everything he wants & shall not let him as long as I can prevent it."[78] Davis was providing both physical and, more important, moral support. Private Fitzpatrick from Georgia, stationed near the crowded Richmond, similarly noted, "The hospitals are overflowing and there is no chance to get [my sick friends] in. The consequence of all this is sad indeed. Jim Webb, I fear, is now dieing and there is 9 chances to one against Stiles Taylor. . . . I moved Stiles to a private house yesterday. . . . I have got straw mattresses for them to lie on and they are fixed up tolerably comfortable."[79] Not only did Fitzpatrick make sure the men were cared for, he acquired the very beds they slept upon. As mentioned earlier, Lt. John Bedingfield did the same for his brothers, acquiring leave to find them hospital space and attend to them when Lewis was shot in the head and Bob languished from dysentery.[80]

Soldiers took responsibility for each other in sickness as surrogates for the prewar care of family members. Comrades were often familiar faces from home, and a man did not want to be reprimanded by one of his fellow soldier's mothers for failing to care for her son in his time of need. When it was a man's own brother or father who fell ill, the stakes were even higher. So the soldiers shared supplies, pooled food in their messes, protected one another from exposure, and made arrangements for the ill—all critical but unspoken soldierly duties.

CIVILIANS AS EDUCATORS AND CARETAKERS

When envisioning the warfront, too often we are tempted to see only soldiers. In fact, soldiers constantly interacted with civilians, relying upon them as conduits of knowledge as well as providers of services and goods that supported health. Those civilians who served as army cooks, launderers, and in other relevant capacities frequently disseminated knowledge on hygiene and environment. Some Confederates, usually officers, were accompanied by their slaves at the warfront, who helped them to accomplish the more mundane aspects of self-care. Further, Virginia residents opened their homes to offer shelter, care, and supplies to soldiers, sometimes even Yankees, especially those who were willing to pay or provide a service in exchange. At times, soldiers found they were uncomfortable relying upon strangers—particularly women and African Americans—but they usually pushed embarrassment aside in favor of survival. Because of the high literacy rates, soldiers also made newspapers part of their civilian network, gleaning recipes, advice, and medical treatments. Even more common, they used correspondence with those at home to provide guidance, psychological support, and supplies. All told, just as the U.S. Sanitary Commission augmented the efficacy of the Union official military medical system, civilians who engaged in the unofficial health care network played frequent and sometimes decisive roles in determining a soldier's fate.

Perhaps the most reliable source of physical civilian aid the soldiers could access were those Americans living or working near the armies. Virginia residents frequently offered food, shelter, and private hospital space. Soldiers praised local care, reminiscent of prewar family care, for its superiority to military treatment. A Confederate artillerist in the Valley wrote that his surgeon gave him permission "to get quarters in a neighboring house" when his throat became so sore he could no longer speak. While there, he received "oil of turpentine externally and internally," which made him "almost well. As soon as the weather clears up, I shall join my company again," he wrote, intimating that bad weather might threaten his fragile health.[81] Shenandoah Valley and Richmond civilians were renowned for their hospitality toward sick Confederates. When the hospitals overflowed with the ailing, many citizens transformed their private residences into convalescent facilities. One Maryland soldier remembered Richmond with some romanticism: "The city . . . had been converted into a huge hospital. The unbounded hospitality of its citizens led them to open their homes to the sick and wounded soldier, and the women were lavish in their attention to the wants of the unfortunate. . . . To the confederate soldier of the Army of Northern Virginia, Richmond will be ever the Mecca enshrined in his heart."[82] Pvt. John O'Farrell agreed that it was "touching indeed, to see the attention paid [the soldiers] by the good ladies of Richmond, hovering around them like angels ministering to their every want," while a Georgian near Richmond found that a plantation overseer took him in when he was too sick to move with "diareah and sick stomach. . . . I can never repay the gratitude I owe to them, I can walk all about now and am determined to take better care of myself this time."[83] Access to home care was most commonly a Confederate benefit, but not in every case.[84] This home advantage, however, was offset by the expansive U.S. Sanitary Commission.

In addition to opening their homes, many civilians living by the warfront outfitted the men with supplies free of charge. Pvt. Henry Handerson of the 9th Louisiana "passed safely through a pretty severe siege of sick-ness and my life is due under Providence to the kindness of Mr Dowe and Mr Newman with whom I am now staying." Handerson further praised "the box of clothing, Mr Dowe kindly brought to me," including "woolen socks," a "jeans coat," and "mittens and comforter."[85] Despite Confederate women's reputation as hostile to Yankees, not every Virginian civilian forsook enemy sufferers. Cpl. Charles F. Read of the 3rd Massachusetts Infantry was on guard duty in the dark and pouring rain with "lightening . . . so vivid that it was almost blinding." A "kind hearted lady living near" took pity and sent out "some bread and coffee, (God bless her for it)."[86] One Jackson foot soldier, in remembering his exhausting march from the Shenandoah Valley campaign to the Peninsula, conjured up "the pleasing sight" of "ladies in white or bright colored dresses," who passed out "baskets of substantial refreshment."[87] Thus Virginian residents, particularly women, made a lasting impression on many soldiers as important components of their self-care networks.

Civilians working for the armies in various capacities also served as vital sources of knowledge about the Virginia environs and as guides to personal care. Some of the most knowledgeable sources of environmental education came from African Americans. Private Fletcher, ever the lice-troubadour, encountered a black laundress in his perpetual quest against persistent pests. He remembered venturing into the hospital laundry and wrote, "It seemed to be run exclusively by women and this did not help my predicament any, as I hated to turn my clothing in even to men. I soon saw who was boss, and I went to her and said in a downcast tone, so none of the others could hear me, that my clothing was lousy and I wished she would have them boiled." Unfortunately, she was not so restrained in her response. "She spoke in a loud tone, and they all heard and laughed: 'Law, child, boiling won't kill them.'"[88] Often Federals would seek out black Virginians, because they tended to be less hostile. Sergeant Ashley and his messmates kept watch on a group of African Americans who were milking cows, only to descend upon them at the choice moment: "[We] all took a good drink and left." Not only did Ashley prey on those he happened across, but he also employed several contrabands to bake nutritious cakes instead of the hardtack he was issued.[89] Some Confederate officers similarly benefited from the presence of one or more slaves from home.[90]

Civilians who remained at home were at least as important to the men's informal network of care as those they encountered near the armies and provided very similar supportive roles. For instance, many men regarded those from their hometowns as sources of continued expertise. Pvt. Charles C. Perkins wrote his local chemist for suggested medicinal remedies when his health became unmanageable in June 1862.[91] Further, many soldiers relied upon correspondence with loved ones to request food and equipment they lacked. Confederate Pvt. David Watson's letter to his mother in Louisa County betrayed a gusto that defied the wintry chill of January. "Dear Mother, The box came to hand on Friday by the wagon that went to Yorktown for provisions with everything safe and in good order." Grateful for the food (in particular, the cake) and the two blankets she had sent, he explained that "it was a great help to my commissary store for I have found foraging around here of late an up-hill business. There are two places here assigned for the country to sell their fowls, eggs, cabbages, & c & there is always a crowd of the Louisianians waiting at each of them to snap up anything that comes along."[92] Some soldiers' lists verged on the absurdly demanding, betraying a frustration with adjusting to the spare life of the soldier. Massachusetts infantryman Lt. Charles Barnard Fox wrote home, "I had better try to have some things which I need very much sent as soon as possible. They are as follows, one nice toaster, to fold to-gether. . . . One small tin coffee-pot, one iron [?] or frying pan . . . one skillet, sauce pan, or small iron kettle, as will pack best" and assorted jugs, bowls, and plates.[93] And yet asking for supplies from home was one of the only options for soldiers who could not afford clothing or food on their sometimes erratic pay.[94]

While letters served as personal supply lines, they were probably most useful for enhancing mental health. Correspondence fostered bravery and steadfastness in the face of environmental adversity, as no soldier wished to appear a coward to his family, and served as continual links to love and family care they remembered from home. The mournful Pvt. Gerald Fitzgerald put it simply: "I hardly know why I take my pen uninspired to write to you unless to provoke an answer for, as I suppose I must have often told you, letters are all I have."[95] A soldier may not have always been cognizant of why he picked up his pen, but once he began his letter, his spirits often lifted. Pvt. Lorenzo Pratt was consumed by homesickness in June in the Valley, but soon after he began writing he felt as though he were home again. "Dear Parantz: as I was sitting in my tent thinking about home and by gone days . . . but I have got no reason to complain."[96] As historian Karen Lystra has explained, Civil War soldiers "experienced certain letters as actual visits of" their correspondents. "When alone they kissed their love letters, carried them to bed, and even spoke to them."[97] Letters were physical talismans that loved ones had touched, providing comfort for soldiers' darkest moments alone in their tents. Sgt. John S. Willey confessed to his wife, "I hav felt so blue ever since [I received your last letter] I though I would not writ untill I felt in better sperrits you can not hav any idea to be placed as I am whare death is starring in our faces and not knowing when this cussed war will end." He admitted his night terrors had become unbearable: "I get so worked up the other nights I could not sleep and grate drops of swett roled of from me."[98] In some cases, men merely wanted validation that their correspondents had some inkling of what they were enduring. Pvt. Henry H. Dedrick explained from the Valley in April, "We are nearly froze. All the balance of my mess is lying down in the tent wrapped up in there blankets. I wish you could see us, then you would say that we had hard times out here."[99] His wife replied, "I tell you Dear Henry my thoughts were fixed on you all them cold snowy days last week. I don't know how you poor fellows can stand it. I know you all have a hard time out there in them cold cotton hats."[100]

For a soldier trapped within the cold walls of the hospital, letters became their real medicine. Such was the case for Sergeant West, who went to the hospital with a dreadfully sore throat. He wrote in his diary that he "was sick all day went to the hospital need a letter from Eliza." Several days later he himself wrote to Eliza to prompt her response.[101] Communicating with a loved one protected West from succumbing to the despair engendered by physical suffering and impersonal care. Unfortunately, many seriously ill soldiers did not have the strength to write home and could not reap the corresponding benefits. Nurses would sometimes write letters on behalf of sick men confined in the hospitals, and Union soldiers could rely upon Sanitary Commission members, but some sick men suffered helplessly. As Pvt. David Bell confessed in a letter with a tone of abject misery, "I had been unwell for five days. I had a pain in mi head and was not fit for duty and did not feel for riting."[102]

Letters were the most intimate conduit home, but soldiers also interacted with civilians via the multitude of newspapers during the Civil War. Newspapers were widely read by the men and thus had the potential to significantly influence health care practices.[103] Some newspapers ran articles on popular remedies, medications, and cooking techniques. Further, certain Union papers provided information on navigating the sprawling infrastructures of the U.S. Medical Department. Yet in 1862, newspapers reported on disease and morale more infrequently than one would suspect given the weightiness of the topics. Reports instead favored battlefield events, wounds, and the progress of generals. The Union papers tended to report on health more often than Confederate papers did, which appeared to reflect pressure from the Sanitary Commission. Indeed, many of the articles addressing health were written by commissioners.

Several articles from the period of the two campaigns did transmit self-care techniques. For instance, the *5th Pennsylvania* printed an excerpt from the *Hall New York Journal of Health*, which held that "in an ordinary camp sickness disables or destroys three times as many as the sword." Its suggestions involved protections from environmental causes of disease, such as wearing certain fabrics—flannel and cotton—and a broad-brimmed hat to prevent sunstroke and avoiding becoming wet to protect against fevers. Drinking water was to be boiled, cooled, and then shaken "so that the oxygen of the air shall get to it."[104] The *Richmond Daily Dispatch* had a suggestion for Confederates that would have been popular with the men: "A small quantity of whiskey twice a day is almost essential to the health of men who undergo such exposures and hardships as those of the soldier." The reporter felt this was particularly true when the men were deprived of coffee, as was the Army of Northern Virginia in 1862.[105] *Harper's Weekly* recommended a solution for muddy, stagnant water: "lemons and liquors . . . to render the water palatable."[106] Incompetent cooking skills were a well-known path to soldier diarrhea, so many newspapers provided the occasional recipe for soldiers to help alleviate the problem.[107] Such recipes often emphasized boiling all ingredients and thoroughly cooking fresh meat. Other articles assessed the health of soldier quarters and sleeping arrangements. One reporter came to the conclusion that the "Sibley tent" was superior to "wedge tents," because it "is conical, and has a chimney-like ventilation." While soldiers had little control over the tents they were issued, they could work to construct a healthier bed. "In point of health, cedar or fir boughs and straw, make the best, if not the safest bed, the soldier can have," explained the same article.[108]

Further, in the Union, which possessed the more bewildering bureaucracy, reporters also helped to illuminate exactly how the military Medical Department was organized, offering some insights for the sick soldier seeking care. Particularly after April 1862, the U.S. Medical Department had undergone a significant reorganization, increasing the number of surgeons and medical staff and the ranks of medical officers. "The medical organization of a regiment consists of a surgeon with an assistant, together with a hospital steward and a dispenser of medicines. There may be other officers, but there are at least these," read an article in the *Christian Recorder*. It then detailed the structures involved in serving the soldiers: "Every regiment has its own hospital, and if a suitable building is not at hand, one or more large tents are furnished for this purpose by the quartermaster." It even equipped the reader to calculate the number of hospitals. "The number of the hospitals in our present army may be estimated by ascertaining the number of regiments and brigades. If five hundred regiments are in the whole field, there will be five hundred hospitals, in addition to the large number of Division and General Hospitals—the latter of which are principally in the cities."[109] While the estimates were overly generous, they did give readers a sense of overall organization and available resources.

THE SEASONED SOLDIER

The men who practiced self-care and built up informal networks of health support advanced toward becoming fully seasoned veterans. Indeed, new insights into this process should help recast our former concepts of seasoning. Soldiers and historians alike have classified wartime seasoning outside of combat as a passive process by which the men contracted, survived, and then became toughened against diseases.[110] While soldiers had little control over the first wave of infectious diseases that pummeled new recruits, they could exert considerable effort to prevent contracting the mental and physical ailments they considered environmental in origin. Yet this is not to suggest that environmental seasoning was somehow more important to becoming a veteran than trial by battle, but rather that environmental seasoning was a more continuous challenge.[111] While the realm of combat contained the greatest horrors of war, it also peculiarly provided a solution for the environmental fixation soldiers developed during the monotony and hardships of camp life. Private Fletcher remembered, "I, with a number of others, had quite an amusing experience—with a happy ending—and it was this: We were suffers from camp diarrhea, as it was called, and up to that time we had found no cure." He continued, "So, entering the battle, I had quite a great fear that something disgraceful might happen and it was somewhat uppermost in my mind; but to my surprise the excitement, or something else, had effected a cure. I inquired of some of the others and they [likewise] reported a cure."[112]

Often the process of environmental seasoning was not entirely conscious until soldiers sensed their own progress and congratulated themselves on becoming "real" soldiers. Capt. Charles M. Blackford of the 5th Alabama Infantry, however, was more vocal about his early failure to adapt. He wrote, "I will fare as the men do and sleep on the ground, as I have been doing ever since the first of March except when sick. This style of life has made me sick and caused all my troubles with dysentery. I hope I will be gradually hardened to it, but when I wake up in the morning cold and wet I am much depressed by it."[113] He sensed that when he became physically "hardened" to such tough living, he would also cease to be so downtrodden. Most men, however, mentioned the positive effects of seasoning once they felt it take hold. Private Blackington wrote home, "I have not had a dry blanket over me for a week or more. I am used to that though. My bones and flesh are as hard and tough as can be and I was never in better health or more rugged than now, notwithstanding stormy weather, hardships, and hard crackers and sometimes not half enough of those." Two weeks later Blackington continued, "I received your letter yesterday afternoon and it found us in good health and spirits. . . . We had a good bit of rain last night and most of us got wet through, but the sun is out this morning and we are fast getting dry. We don't mind a wetting now anymore than a lot of ducks would."[114] And Captain Morgan recalled soldier seasoning in this way in his memoir: "How did we stand those long, tiresome marches, through the rain and the mud of spring, through the dust and heat of summer, and midst snow and ice of winter, often poorly shod, scantily clothed, and on short, very short rations. . . . It took men to do these things—men with muscles, sinews, and nerves in their bodies, and courage in their hearts; and then, on the battlefield to meet the foe."[115] As both soldiers revealed, men took pride in their evolution, whether as an enlisted man or an officer.

At an earlier point in his soldier career, Pvt. Edward A. Moore from Maryland might have been extremely bothered by the "most wretched weather, real winter again, rain or snow almost all the time" in the Valley. But instead he had acclimated: "One night about midnight I was awakened by hearing a horse splashing through the water just outside of the tent and a voice calling to the inmates to get out of the flood. . . . My bunk was on a little rise. I put my hand out—into the water. I determined, however, to stay as long as I could, and was soon asleep, which showed that I was becoming a soldier."[116] Equally important to his physical ability to withstand the rain was his determination to sleep at all costs. Private Worsham was a Jackson infantryman, who departed the grueling Valley campaign only to end up in Richmond for the Seven Days. After getting his first real rest since April—a day off to enjoy the city—he commented, "We left Richmond a year ago in new uniforms, with the fair complexion of city men. . . . We returned now ruddy and brown with the health and hardness that outdoor living creates, and we were veterans."[117] Finally, Sergeant Pryor noted that seasoning marked a man's transition from civilian to soldier, contributing to the disdain veterans sometimes espoused about green recruits. "Our time for camp sickness is past. We are just as healthy here now as weed be at home. It dont hurt us to do without sleep or to get wet & dry without changing clothes. Wee can now stand the service, those of us that have passed through the fiery ordeal of becoming climatized & accostomed to camp life." But he noted, "The recruits fare badly."[118] Progressing to veteran status was highly gratifying, and yet it was also a reminder that soldiers had shed an integral part of their former identities. As much as they valued correspondence as a means to explain their transformation, they were now irreversibly different from those at home.

While common soldiers and their officers could agree that a seasoned soldier was a more valuable commodity than a fresh recruit, commanders proved hostile toward the means by which soldiers acquired environmental seasoning. Within the context of military structure, individual volition was not necessarily something to be celebrated. Indeed, in order to successfully practice many of the self-care techniques described, from foraging to locating clean water, soldiers often had to straggle. Further, it is quite clear from soldier accounts that straggling itself became one of the most popular ways to relieve the strain of environmental hardships, receive home-quality care for disease, and revive falling spirits. In short, straggling both enabled self-care and was a self-care technique of paramount importance in 1862 when the military medical systems were still being constructed. Thus a tension was set up: soldiers needed to take care of themselves—commanders expected them to—and yet the men would occasionally have to bend the rules of discipline to achieve their health goals.

5

Straggling and the Limits of Self-Care

The regimentation of military life was intended to deny individuality. In doing so, it aimed to fortify mental health by serving as a barrier against inaction, resignation, and reluctance to kill and physical health by regulating camp behavior and hygiene. It compelled soldiers to complete the mundane and unpalatable duties necessary to maintaining an army, typically a source of disgruntlement for volunteers. It also, however, handcuffed soldiers to simplistic procedures in highly complex situations and could, contradictorily, engender passivity, as some men were tempted to forfeit responsibility for their survival up the chain of command. Herein lay the paradox of self-care. Self-care required individuality, reliance on a network of care outside of formal army structures, and, most of all, straggling. In short, self-care ran counter to the tenets of military discipline, but in 1862 it also better served soldier health than did the medical systems.[1] While there were many other reasons to straggle, soldiers who self-identified as straggling in pursuit of health did not see themselves as lacking devotion to cause.[2] They believed they were exemplary soldiers who did not stray because they were weak or cowardly, but in order to return to the ranks healthier and in better spirits. They identified as seasoned veterans who knew how to extract their best chances for survival.

Commanders, on the contrary, did not parse the various motivations behind absenteeism, nor did they recognize self-care as legitimate. They saw instead the typical unwillingness of citizen soldiers to assimilate into military life and bear up under its hardships.[3] As the numbers of those present in the ranks dwindled for a variety of reasons, commanders justifiably believed their armies to be dangerously vulnerable to enemy attack.

While they initially recognized that logistical complications contributed to straggling, when conditions began to improve they resolved to terminate what they considered the associated disciplinary problem.[4] Thus, generals increasingly reprimanded stragglers, placing limitations on self-care as 1862 wore on. While subordinate officers tended to remain more sympathetic to their soldiers' plights, and some War Department officials pushed for furloughs as an antidote for straggling, the command interpretation of the problem and solution won the day. After all, solving straggling by constricting punishment—even associating it with desertion and the corresponding death penalty—was simpler than getting to the complex roots of continued sickness and demoralization. By the end of the year, commanders had at least partially succeeded in forcing soldiers back into the paternalistic medical system, which served military goals and not necessarily the individual's will to survive.

Straggling is defined as being absent from camp or roll call without leave, as every enlisted man who wished to leave the ranks was required to obtain a pass from his commander. One of the most common disciplinary infractions of the war, straggling was distinct from desertion—a permanent withdrawal from the ranks without permission—in that it was the soldier's intent to return to his unit after a temporary hiatus, be it several hours or several weeks.[5] Soldiers straggled for many reasons, some of which overlapped with reasons for desertion, but only two reasons are relevant to self-care: first, straggling for relief from environmental strain (which soldiers feared might lead to sickness and diminished spirits), and second, straggling to pursue self-care techniques, such as locating clean water or berries, or seeking civilian home care.[6] This is not to suggest that no stragglers were feigning illness but rather to reframe certain types of absenteeism as what might be termed strategic straggling. Historians have often conflated straggling and desertion in their studies, because of some overlapping soldier motivations and because, as historian Mark Weitz explains, "Straggling and desertion were essentially the same in that they depleted the army of manpower."[7] While Weitz is unquestionably correct that in the immediate sense stragglers were not available for roll call (which was also command's main objection), strategic straggling counteracts this argument. Some men who fell back in pursuit of self-care could recover sufficiently to resume duty as effective soldiers, whereas if they had remained in the ranks they might have deteriorated or even died.

Another reason that exploring straggling as distinct from desertion has been so difficult for scholars is that soldiers were justifiably reticent about

enteeism in their letters and diaries, while generals' interpre-
much easier to come by. Common soldiers not only feared being
by officers and punished, but they also feared the stigma of
—a crushing blow to reputation that can be difficult for modern
s to comprehend. As historian Gerald Linderman has explored,
cowardice was considered "the one sin which may not be pardoned either
in this world or the next."[8] Thus, direct references to straggling in eyewitness accounts are relatively rare, though a careful combing of the evidence
reveals likely episodes. These accounts must be augmented with memoirs,
because soldiers proved more likely to admit to disciplinary infractions
when they could justify their actions at length without fear of retribution.
Memoirs can be misleading, but it is safe to say that soldiers who returned
to the ranks without compulsion were stragglers, not deserters. In the end,
as problematic as these sources are for investigating soldier motivations
behind absenteeism, if we take soldiers at their words, improving health
and spirits and avoiding environmental hardships were major reasons to
straggle in 1862. This type of straggling demands separate consideration
from desertion, because it could improve soldier performance, even if it
depleted armies in the short term.

THE ART OF STRATEGIC STRAGGLING

Pvt. Henry E. Handerson of the 9th Louisiana reflected in his memoirs
upon an incident from March 11, 1862. "The rain had fallen almost inces-
santly during our march, and our camps . . . were converted into shallow
lakes by the standing water, which prevented comfortable rest by night
or day. After a week or more of such experience, thoroughly worn out by
want of sleep, I determined one rainy evening to slip quietly out of camp
and seek some shelter where I might rest comfortably for one night at
least." Though treading lightly in his memoirs for the sake of his children
(his intended audience), Handerson's euphemism is clear: the private was
straggling. Not wishing to appear a coward, he explained, "I felt desperate enough to face almost anything for the chance of securing shelter."
Handerson knew that if caught, he could face a number of humiliating
punishments as a straggler or, worse yet, be falsely accused of desertion,
court-martialed, and executed. But desperation was born of experience.
The previous October, he had suffered a prolonged bout of typhoid fever,
resulting in weeks at a Charlottesville hospital and subsequent convalescence in a civilian home. By March, he was with his unit but serving in a
reduced capacity—as the captain's bookkeeper—to preserve his strength.[9]

Like other common soldiers, he believed exposing himself to rain might renew his sickness, and so he fled the ranks.

Handerson's quest for reprieve from the elements eventually led him to a church. "Opening the door carefully and peering within, a novel sight met my eye. Most of the pews were already occupied by soldiers who had fled to the sacred building for shelter, each of them having preempted his own position and spread his blanket upon the seat." To add to the gathering's comfort, "A large fire had been started in the stove, upon the surface of which numerous slices of bacon were cooking and diffusing an appetizing odor throughout the building." Handerson curled up to sleep, but "in the morning, refreshed and strengthened by a comfortable night's rest, I returned to my command, where, so far as I know, I had not been missed."[10] What Handerson discovered was that in the midst of a storm, scores of soldiers stole away from camp to seek proper shelter, where they could cook, eat a hot meal, and recover. The next morning, to the private's recollection (or, at least, admission), he promptly returned to the ranks.

One of the most common reasons soldiers cited for straggling was indeed excessive exposure to extreme weather. As Private McKim remembered, veterans recognized when environmental strain became too much to bear, such as in spring 1862 in the Shenandoah Valley: "When we had no tents and when the weather was so inclement and our exposure so unusually severe, we would slip off to some private house whenever opportunity offered and leave could be obtained, and sometimes without leave. Only in this way, I think, could we have endured the ordeal."[11] McKim enjoyed the Confederate benefit of being warmly welcomed into Shenandoah Valley homes, while Union soldiers more often sought solace in churches and barns. But that is not to say that no Union soldiers were invited into Southern homes. Private Wood was a Massachusetts man in the Valley who straggled in search of water to a civilian house on an exceedingly hot day ("it was 'said' that the thermometer yesterday in the shade stood at a hundred and ten degrees"). Residents obliged him, and as a thank-you he mended their broken clock, since in civilian life he had been a clock-maker. Later Wood also visited a friend in the Valley, Miss Vowell, who promised to nurse him if he ever fell ill.[12] It is important to bear in mind, however, that Union soldiers were often straggling in hostile territory and took some risk when they approached civilians in private homes.

While these cases of straggling tended to be based on individual whims, at times a particularly grueling march would devolve into mass straggling. On a painfully hot day in August on the Peninsula, a Massachusetts artilleryman, Pvt. E. Kendall Jenkins, explained, "Hundreds 'fell out' some died. Glass told 106 [degrees] in shade."[13] When enormous dust clouds choked Confederates on the road near Malvern Hill back in July, Pvt. Kinchen Carpenter from North Carolina wrote that "many of the soldiers stayed behind, lay down in the woods and did not get with their command until next day and, I, one of them. Under strict military rules this was an offense and no doubt many an officer would have put some hardship on us for doing so."[14] The soldiers realized they could be punished but were too desperate to care. Confederate Pvt. William R. Smith managed to keep in the ranks himself but could hardly blame his comrades for straggling, considering the snow storm pummeling them in April: "After a hard days march arrived here near dark with a few stragglers more than half of the boys left along the road having given out. I stood it though I was very tired."[15] By then the snow was several inches deep.

Mud was one of the most common environmental factors to prompt straggling, because it made sleeping in camp unpleasant and impaired one's ability to keep up on the march. One night, Cpl. Horace M. Wade of the 12th Virginia Cavalry tried sleeping on rails with just his coat to protect himself from the muddy ground during a deluge. He fared poorly. The following evening, he slipped off into the woods to locate a broad-canopied tree, which provided a vastly superior night's sleep.[16] Private Patterson of the 9th Alabama appeared to have little choice but to straggle given his regiment's experience near Lebanon Church, Virginia. He wrote of a march that "beggars description. The night was so dark that it was absolutely impossible to see anything and we relied entirely on the sense of hearing and feeling." It was not the dark so much as the rain that afflicted the men. "And the mud and water was literally knee deep, and the men would run against each other, strike their faces against another's back or gun without seeing anything." The result was almost comical. "Some fell in mudholes and had to be dragged out, and our regiment became scattered for a mile, and all along the road you could hear, 'This way, Co. D,' 'Hear is your company A,' 'Close up Company C,' &c &c." Patterson did what he could to keep up. "I continued the march about 5 miles when I ran into a clump of bushes, and winding myself up in my wet blankets as well as I could remained there until daylight, keeping the bushes under me as much as possible to keep from drowning."[17] He found his comrades in the morning, one of whom complained that he had lost his boots in the quagmire. Though Patterson was only gone a few hours, technically he had strayed from the ranks. In a similar situation, Private Handerson explained that numerous men had been separated from their units in the rain and dark one night. "The rain was still falling dismally as, wet cold and hungry, we endeavored to retrace our steps of the preceding day. . . . As we progressed towards our supposed rear we overtook numerous stragglers, bent, like ourselves, on finding their commands."[18] These men captured the chaos of soldiering that could result in what was essentially unintentional straggling.[19]

A related reason soldiers straggled was because of illness. Because they believed exposure to the environment of war had contributed to their sickness, they sought protection in the form of shelter, while some went further to seek civilian home care. In Confederate Pvt. William C. McClellan's case, he believed that mud undid his fragile health. "We had 10 miles to march and a Bad Road. We started in a few minutes it was so dark We could not see our hands before us and then I would fall into a mud hole up to my knees." As a result, "I have a very violent cold some fever." He cast off restraint and made for the nearest civilian quarters. An industrious Southerner welcomed McClellan and fellow absentees into his home for the price of one dollar each, providing "a glorious nights rest" on the carpet. Though still a bit unwell when he returned to the ranks the next morning, McClellan was glad to have spent the height of his fever in front of a roaring fire.[20] Lt. Elisha F. Paxton, a Virginian, also fell sick and informally quit the ranks to stay in a nearby civilian house. "The weather is worse upon us than last winter," he wrote home. "Then the ground was frozen and we had the satisfaction at least of being dry—having dry clothes and dry blankets. But now everything is wet and we have no tents. It has had no happy effect upon my health. Yesterday I left the brigade to stay in a house a few days, but think I shall join it again to-morrow."[21] Paxton waited for the worst of the wet weather to pass to prevent himself from becoming seriously ill. Pvt. Charles Perkins was one of the rare soldiers, who practiced a varied self-care regimen but remained very ill for nearly the entire year with diarrhea, rheumatism, and "bilious afflictions." His routines involved occasionally straggling for relief to a "chateau." At other points in the year, he kept falling out of the ranks because of leg pains or stayed behind in his tent with a wet cloth on his forehead.[22]

Other soldiers chose to straggle when their spirits suffered from exposure and sickness. Henry Keiser described not one but three separate instances of straggling on the Peninsula after feeling "played out," a phrase referring to physical exhaustion and mental resignation.[23] Sgt. William West of the 6th Maine was hospitalized for typhoid fever in early 1862, and, after rejoining his unit, his once jubilant pride in soldiering dissipated into sadness. In spring on the march, he "had to fall out and go back to the camp." West stayed behind all day and night with no permission, lamenting that he felt "real home-sick." One month later in April, he remained troubled by illness and straggled again. "I being sick fell out and joined the wagons. I lay alongside of the road for an hour in the woods very sick joined the wagon trains when they came along. did not join the regt but Bill Merritt & I camped along side of the road."[24] West's transformation to troubled soldier was stark. It was also a serious problem for his unit, as noncommissioned officers like West played significant roles in encouraging the rank and file.

Returning to some of the earlier stories in which soldiers practiced self-care, it is apparent that many techniques required straggling to execute. At close reading, Pvt. William Stilwell's story about washing his clothes to improve mental and physical health very likely included straggling. He noted that "we went about half mile from camp, pulled off stark naked and went out to wash like good fellows, dried and put them on again."[25] Pvt. Jacob Blackington and his messmate Jake on the Peninsula almost surely straggled in their quest to provide themselves with ample quantities of swamp berries on their Peninsula marches.[26] Private Wood was also adept at stealing off to locate cherries and apples to maintain his solid health and cheerful countenance.[27] Nearly any of the self-care techniques—locating clean water, seeking additional exercise, searching out medicinal roots—could prompt a temporary abandonment of the ranks. Most of the soldiers' self-care goals, besides seeking shelter, only consumed their attention for several hours at a time, but even their brief straggling contributed to an overall appearance of disciplinary chaos that concerned commanders and sometimes attracted public ridicule.

Cavalrymen found it easiest to straggle in pursuit of self-care, as they enjoyed the benefit of being on horseback.[28] Cavalryman Ashley from New York wrote boldly of "foraging for my own benefit, and patroling for my own satisfaction, my duties in camp are finished about 11 O'Clock then I am at liberty to stroll; within 4 days I have picked upwards of 20 quarts of beautiful Blackberries which will make a good relish."[29] While he may very well have had free time, Ashley's near constant adventures outside the ranks suggest that he could have easily been construed as a straggler. When combined with the benefit of being stationed near their families, as in the case of Stonewall Jackson's troopers, cavalrymen tended to straggle for longer periods—known as the French Furlough—which could last weeks (though they seldom wrote their own accounts of these visitations). Typically, the cavalry are portrayed by historians as leaving the ranks to tend to farm and family, which was indeed on their minds.[30] But straggling was much easier for troopers to justify to themselves given the miserable environmental conditions they endured and their frequent illnesses. Yet it wasn't only Jackson's cavalrymen who took advantage of being close to home to straggle; many of his foot soldiers disappeared for days or weeks, especially in the inclement winter and early spring.[31]

It was officers' jobs to keep such sick, underequipped, and suffering men in the ranks, which they found increasingly difficult to rationalize, especially when they, too, took to falling out without orders. Michigan infantryman Lieutenant Haydon managed to keep to his duties: "It is no exaggeration to say that I was many times in the main road in mud to my knees. It required great exertion to urge on the men & keep them in the ranks."[32] Knee-deep in muck, he felt great sympathy for his men, while officers higher up the chain of command tended to be more critical. For instance, after the battle of Williamsburg, Maj. Gen. D. H. Hill noted that "thousands of soldiers had sought shelter from the storm of the night before in barns and outhouses, and it was with the utmost difficulty they could be driven out. Cold, tired, hungry, and jaded, many seemed indifferent alike to life or capture."[33] Hill portrayed the men as unequal to the rigors of their job, when soldiers reported that straggling was instead their attempt to persevere.

For the most part, officers enjoyed less rigorous physical demands as befit their ranks, creating some distance between themselves and common soldiers, but also producing feelings of sympathy and guilt. While officers were supposed to sleep by their men in camp unless given specific permission to seek other quarters, they enjoyed more freedom and less potential punishment than enlisted men.[34] Lt. Elisha F. Paxton complained about the effects the wet was having on his health and wrote, "Yesterday I left the brigade to stay in a house a few days, but think I shall join it again tomorrow."[35] Maj. Frank B. Jones suffered from heat with a violent headache and "felt depressed and miserable." First he slipped out of the ranks for a "pleasant" nap "under an apple tree." That night as his "men bivouacked on the wet ground," he "was fortunate enough to get into a carpenter shop and slept comfortably on the dry floor."[36] In such cases, the officers were modeling loose discipline by example and thus proved less critical of their own stragglers. For instance, when Pvt. John Casler stole off in search of whiskey to revive his spirits and was reported to his superior, the officer just laughed and looked the other way. Casler was not so lucky later in the year when stragglers were targeted for increased punishment. That incident resulted in Casler being bucked and gagged (binding one's arms and slipping them over one's knees, while gagging the mouth with a bayonet) from sun up to sun down, almost prompting him to desert.[37]

Overall, soldiers who straggled for self-care believed that absenteeism was simply par for the course in soldier life. They were not receiving proper protection from exposure in the ranks, nor were they obtaining the health care they desired. It was not that they had failed to acculturate into the army. Junior officers also often recognized why the men were straggling and even took their own informal leaves for similar reasons. When viewed from inside the ranks, these spontaneous acts of defiance appeared reasonable, but from the command perspective, the armies had fallen into a dangerous state of disorder.

COMMANDERS AND THE LIMITS OF SELF-CARE

The reports on straggling in 1862 confirm that the net effect of absenteeism was indeed potentially devastating to the armies. Straggling occurred during the campaigns for many reasons, including logistical problems, command errors, and poor guides, and only some of the mass straggling was conducted in order to achieve self-care. And yet, command saw all straggling as disarray. Hence as the year wore on, leaders became increasingly intolerant of the offense. Early on, army regulations stipulated no particular chastisement, and so officers doled out penalties as they saw fit—usually fairly minor in scope—often meant to humiliate and prove unpleasant rather than severely punish. A soldier's penance might include being forced to ride a "wooden horse," don a "barrel shirt," dig latrines, bury dead horses, or forfeit pay for the period of one's absence.[38] While historian Ella Lonn claimed that Confederate officers were "more ingenious with their barrel-jackets, gagging, and bucking, probably because they were more loath to lose [scarce] men by inflicting the full rigor of the law," illustrations of camp punishments by the Union's Private Billings suggest that Federals also encountered an inspired assortment of reprimands. But as Lonn points out, "In the end both [Federals and Confederates] had to come to exacting the death penalty"; this was indeed the direction commanders were heading in 1862 as frustration mounted.[39] By the end of the year, it had become distinctly more dangerous for soldiers to attempt self-care if it required straggling and might be construed as desertion.

The most dramatic battle over straggling in 1862 Virginia, and certainly the best documented, occurred in Stonewall Jackson's army. Indeed, the story of Jackson's men best demonstrates the hardening of commanders' attitudes toward straggling, because the offense was pervasive in his ranks with some regiments losing over twenty percent of their forces.[40] Because an unusual number of Jackson's men were stationed close by their families, many of them were gone for weeks as they recovered at home.

In the winter of 1861 to 1862, Jackson refused to rest his men by grant-ing furloughs; instead, he drilled them until he received permission to pursue his Romney campaign. As discussed earlier, the campaign was a bitter January endeavor both in weather and in lack of significant strategic gains. Pvt. Charles W. Trueheart, an artillerist, provided a stark portrait: "The roads were so slippery with sleet, that the poor [horses] could not keep their feet in pulling the cannon & wagons, but fell continually— sometimes 3 out of 4 of a team would be down at once. Splotches and puddles of blood frequently marked the places where they fell. . . . Many of us got our feet and hands frostbitten. My feet were so badly bitten that I could scarcely walk."[41] The soldiers faced freezing temperatures on the march and when they reached Romney had nowhere to sleep. Historian Peter Cozzens writes, "The men took it upon themselves to find shelter" in private houses, churches, and stores.[42] That winter, Col. Turner Ashby's cavalry became particularly notorious for employing the lengthier French Furlough, sometimes for up to four weeks. Such extended stays were risky, as they smacked of permanence, alerting commanders to the prospect of desertion. As Lt. Albert C. Lincoln, a subordinate of Ashby, fretted on February 18, 1862, "That portion of the [7th Virginia Cavalry] that are now at home have left three or four times in the same manner. . . . Some of them had not been back more than three weeks since the retreat from Romney."[43]

By the time the Shenandoah Valley campaign commenced in March, Jackson's men had a reputation for straggling. Then, on April 16, 1862, the Confederate Congress passed the Conscript Act, which among other stipu-lations required all one-year enlistees from 1861 to remain in uniform for two more years.[44] There is some debate among scholars as to whether the first national draft in history discouraged or encouraged desertion.[45] Conscription probably made little difference to strategic straggling, which was not about commitment to the stars and bars but rather one's personal survival. There was, however, evident hostility toward the draft in the Val-ley, where cannoneer Pvt. Edward A. Moore recalled his fellow Confed-erate 1st Marylanders resisting the reelection of their officers in protest. Moore's account made clear that the men were not lazy or unpatriotic. They had faced hard times in "wretched" camps, marches in mud "up to their knees," "severe weather" and snow up "through March and far into April," treks back and forth over the mountains, which amounted to "two months of marching and countermarching, without any object that we could divine, under conditions of more acute discomfort than we had ever known before." Moore remembered Stonewall Jackson as starkly callous, explaining that when one agonized Marylander cursed the general, Jackson overheard and barked, "It's for your own good, sir!"[46] While the story's veracity is questionable, one effect of conscription was indeed that Jackson focused his scrutiny more acutely upon any man who strayed from the ranks, because manpower had become such a pressing concern.

Meanwhile the general continued to enforce an exhausting marching pace across mountain passes that pushed his men to their physicals limits. In April, Sgt. McHenry Howard noted, "We were eating on the porch of [a] house, which was close by the side of the Turnpike, some time in the afternoon, when . . . wagons and ambulances soon came hurrying past to the rear. With them there were a number of stragglers." The absentees latched onto the medical wagons, and superiors surmised that they might be malingering. Howard reported that his commander, Brig. Gen. Charles S. Winder, remarked, "That must be stopped," with no discussion as to why the straggling might have arisen.[47] By June, Jackson's army appeared to some observers to be self-destructing from exhaustion and exposure. Confederate stragglers scattered the Valley Turnpike, being plucked up by Federals as prisoners of war.[48]

Four hundred miles of active campaigning later, Jackson's "foot cavalry" disembarked from the Valley on June 17 for the Peninsula and scarcely paused again until July 8. By then "some of the men had not washed their hands and faces for five or six days."[49] Sanitation gravely suffered, and men were sick as dogs. Desertion and straggling spiked once more.[50] As Pvt. John H. Worsham explained, much of the straggling was simply from exhaustion. The private "sat down in a little fence corner to get some rest" and, after tending to a sick comrade, "fell asleep, and did not wake till morning."[51] The army Jackson was joining for the Seven Days campaign was hardly free of absenteeism itself.

That June, when Lee assumed command of the soon-to-be-christened Army of Northern Virginia, he could scarcely believe its disorder. The Seven Days battles were imperiled by straggling for a number of reasons, only some of which had to do with self-care. Brig. Gen. John B. Magruder could put only 7,100 of his 12,500 infantry and two of his sixteen batteries into battle on July 1 at Malvern Hill. As historian Stephen Sears wrote, "Every road and every grove behind Magruder's front was filled with his stragglers."[52] The problem was hardly isolated to Magruder's troops. Stationed near Richmond on July 1, the army disintegrated into "hordes of stragglers [turning] the city into a veritable resort town." Local newspapers lambasted army discipline, calling for the death penalty. Approximately fifty stragglers per day were arrested in Staunton in the month of July as they poured in from the east.[53] The addition of Jackson's troops from the Valley worsened matters, as his exhausted men refused orders, and Jackson himself fell asleep for a major part of the action.[54] Historian Joseph Harsh has provided detailed evidence that by August and September 1862, Lee became obsessed with identifying and punishing stragglers, rebuking them as the "cowards of the army."[55] Lee also wrote to President Davis in September of the need for more legislation and punishment regarding the offense.[56]

Though Jackson censured one of his own, General Winder, for bucking and gagging his absentees, considering it not a useful deterrent, Jackson eventually took a far harder stance against the disciplinary infraction.[57] In August, he executed four deserters, some of whom argued that they had only been straggling.[58] Command complaints to the Confederacy's War Department had, in the meantime, prompted Adj. Gen. Samuel Cooper to take his own actions of increasing severity. He first issued General Order 16 on March 21, 1862, abolishing furloughs for men except those on medical leave. By May, he added Special Order 107, arresting all absentees for prompt court-martial. If stragglers refused arrest, they would be automatically punished as deserters: death by firing squad. Secretary of State George W. Randolph pleaded with the governors of the various Rebel states on July 17, 1862, to do their part in rounding up stragglers and deserters: "Our armies are so much weakened by desertions, and by the absence of officers and men without leave, that we are unable to reap the fruits of our victories. . . . We have resorted to courts-martial and military executions, and we have ordered all officers employed in enrolling conscripts to arrest both deserters and absentees, and offered rewards for the former."[59] In August, General Order 94 called for extreme policing of the rear on any march: "On all marches a Division Provost Marshal, with a guard of one commissioned and two non-commissioned officers and ten men from each regiment will march in rear of each division, accompanied by one of the Division Medical officers, to prevent straggling." Further, "When men fall back who are sick, the Surgeon will give them a ticket for transportation in the ambulances or train of wagons. If not sick they will be marched into camp under charge of the guard."[60] By December, Confederate General Order 137 institutionalized a slew of new convictions for stragglers and deserters, ranging from strapping a twelve-pound iron to one's legs, forfeiting an entire year of pay, and receiving lashes.[61] There is evidence to suggest these more strident measures did help to tighten discipline and reduce straggling after 1862.[62]

Straggling in the Union armies in 1862 Virginia was also a considerable problem, though Federals did not often have the temptation of being close to their families, as did some units from Virginia. Union straggling in the Valley was pervasive because the armies were frightfully limited in rations, equipment, and medical supplies. *Frank Leslie's Illustrated Newspaper* famously pictured General Frémont's army as "ragged," hunched, and straggling as a result of poor conditions.[63] Brig. Gen. Louis Blenker's division was gaining a reputation for both straggling and plundering, because they had long been without "tents, shelter, or knapsacks" and without pay since December. General Frémont drew considerable criticism for failing to reign in Blenker's "Dutch vandals." In Shield's division, one 110th Pennsylvanian committed suicide from exhaustion on March 21, while only one in five of his comrades reported present for duty. April discipline was likewise lax, as the men continued to trickle away in search of much-needed supplies and shelter. Shields complained to Banks that he had had to arrest Col. George H. Gordon's men from the 3rd Wisconsin and 2nd Massachusetts, who had been "loitering" around Edinburg. Gordon gruffly countered in a letter that his men had been foraging because of a severe lack of rations, attempting to draw attention to the source rather than the result of the problem to little effect. June brought more physical torment and, thus, more straggling. Shields's men were at half rations, prompting the army to act as "a marauding party, plundering everyone."[64]

The Peninsula campaign, being the larger, more important endeavor, drew more attention from U.S. officials on the topic of discipline. Charles Tripler, the U.S. Peninsula medical director, complained, "Whenever a march was undertaken straggling was permitted to go on unrestrained, and I fear was sometimes even encouraged by officers whose duty it was to have prevented it." As the director implied, upper-level command often blamed regimental officers for allowing the straggling to go unchecked. Tripler even witnessed soldiers charging the hospital boats to flee the field, leading him to announce, "I . . . determined to send no more men from the Peninsula on account of sickness if there were any means of avoiding it."[65] Partially as a means to curb straggling, McClellan issued a new whiskey ration in mid-May, but this paltry nod to the men's comfort had limited effect.[66] McClellan, too, grew increasingly impatient with what he interpreted as malingering and shirking of duty. "Absentees tell such exaggerated stories of the hardships and sufferings of campaign life . . . that they deter troops from enlisting. . . . There are two well men absent to one really sick man."[67]

The Seven Days battles did not improve matters for the Army of the Potomac. Following the Union victory at Malvern's Hill, the general ordered an eight-mile retreat to Harrison's Landing that resulted in significant

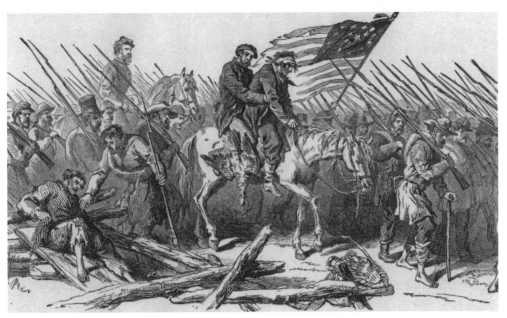

*"The Army of General Fremont on Its March up the Shenandoah Valley—
Wounded and Ragged Soldiers"* (Frank Leslie's Illustrated Newspaper,
War Supplement, *July 5, 1862*)

Union absenteeism. Rain pummeled the exhausted Federals for twenty-four hours. Historian Sears writes, "Something about this downpour seemed the last straw, seemed to wash away the bonds that had held the army together." Men tossed off their weapons, and most of the 818 men listed as missing from the preceding battle were collected as absentees rather than on the battlefield. U.S. cavalry regulars rounded up nearly 1,200 stragglers in the rear.[68] July in Harrison's Landing—a lengthy hiatus in the alternating heat and rain with little to do—did not help matters. Individual regimental records show that men deserted or strayed from the ranks in striking numbers because of the poor conditions.[69]

By July 13, President Lincoln took notice of the mass absenteeism in McClellan's ranks. Lincoln warned, "45,000 of your Army [are] still alive, and not with it. I believe half, or two thirds of them are fit for duty to-day. . . . How can they be got to you? and how can they be prevented from getting away in such numbers for the future?" While McClellan haggled with Lincoln's numbers, he admitted, "The number . . . really absent is thirty eight thousand two hundred fifty. . . . I quite agree with you that more than one half these men are probably fit for duty to-day. I have frequently called the attention lately of the War Dept to the evil of absenteeism." But he had hope that he could curb the problem at Harrison's Landing: "Leakages by desertion occur in every Army and will occur here of course, but I do not at all . . . anticipate anything like a recurrence of what has taken place."[70] Contrary to McClellan's prediction, straggling continued. McClellan passed on responsibility to officials in Washington and it would be left to his successor, Ambrose E. Burnside, to improve some of the logistical problems underlying straggling.[71]

The United States took longer to implement a slightly less punitive approach to absenteeism than did the Confederacy, in part because of an advantage in manpower and also because Lincoln favored moderation to appease a scrutinizing public. The August U.S. General Order Number 18 required that all commanders of regiments and companies march continually in the rear collecting absentees. There was only one excuse for a laggard: "written permit from the medical officer of the regiment that they are too sick to perform the march, and therefore must ride in ambulances."[72] This put the walking sick in considerable peril. The order also made little progress on correcting the offense, and Lincoln continued to survey the problem from the capital, urging McClellan to action. He was aghast that those on furlough together with those absent from the ranks without permission outnumbered the new recruits. But Lincoln also remained reluctant to conflate straggling and desertion, fearing public backlash to the army's practice of capital punishment.[73] Americans had historically criticized military discipline deemed too harsh, and Lincoln critically needed public support of the war effort, especially given the impending change of war aims to include emancipation.

Under considerable pressure from the respective War Departments, commanders on both sides, in turn, put pressure on their Medical Departments to eliminate straggling by scrutinizing the sick. Surgeons were instructed to be skeptical of illness that lacked overt symptoms as potential cases of malingering. In this vein, Confederate Surgeon General Moore warned his surgeons "that the pains of Chronic Rheumatism are easily feigned and that Medical officers should be very careful in their examinations of such cases, and approve of the discharge of such as show in their person, evident marks of this disease."[74] No doubt, some soldiers feigned illness to escape their duties; however, many soldiers complained of being increasingly turned away from morning sick call without care. Slow-developing diseases, such as scurvy, which took months to manifest, were marked by a gradual onslaught of debilitating aches and pains, in addition to depressed spirits. In short, diseases could easily be missed or misdiagnosed. In another misguided interpretation of the situation,

Tripler appeared to believe that healthy soldiers were straggling away from the ranks only to succumb to illness outside the care and comfort of army infrastructures: "Hundreds were collected in the woods and in houses and huts and in our old position at Camp Winfield Scott who were borne not upon the surgeon's reports." The stragglers were allegedly brought in "after days of privation had brought on actual disease."[75] It is far more likely that the men had straggled because of illness or fear of falling sick in the first place.

In short, high command and their medical directors began to devote an increasing amount of energy to punishing absenteeism over the course of 1862, eventually addressing only the logistical aspect of the problem and then only months after the two campaigns of the study. Leaders categorized the majority of straggling as malingering or cowardice and even began to conflate the problem with desertion. There were a number of reasons for this hardline stance, some of which have already been raised. Generals expected volunteers to buck discipline and took their straggling as confirmation of what was a common critique of citizen soldiers at the time. Further, though generals recognized that their men were suffering, they believed that suffering was part of the soldier job description and should be borne with courage, as befit their class values. Additionally, if commanders tried to get to the bottom of the strategic straggling, they would be opening a Pandora's box of trouble, involving issues that were not within their capacities to rectify, such as limited medical knowledge. Finally, and perhaps most important, a commanding general had a different role in waging war than did a common soldier. Generals shouldered the weighty responsibility for winning battles and needed a critical number of men present in the ranks to accomplish their plans. This was McClellan's persistent refrain during the Peninsula campaign.[76] Commanders had to contend with the impatience of the public and the civilian demand for tactical victories, especially in the eastern theater, which was vital to keeping the war effort going. While commanders had to absolve the confirmed sick of their duties, they clung desperately to the seemingly able-bodied men who remained in the ranks, even if those men were breaking down.

THE FURLOUGH AS MISSED OPPORTUNITY

There was one officially sanctioned method of preventing strategic straggling: the furlough or leave of absence. Rest and removal not only from combat but also from the grueling routines of camp life was often the best chance for a soldier to recover from malaise and illness.[77] The absence also allowed time for soldiers to reconnect with friends and family and attend to important matters back home, bolstering spirits and curbing all sources of straggling, not just self-care. Yet furloughs were a contentious issue in 1862 and remained so throughout a war troubled by a shortage of manpower. The Confederate and Union War Departments were willing to hold out thirty- or even sixty-day furloughs as carrots for reenlistment, while generals often complained that these policies deprived them of critical mass.[78]

The Confederate conversation about furloughs in 1862 is particularly instructive as to why some officials and regimental officers favored this alternative and generals tended to resist it. The Confederate War Department issued General Order 1 on January 1, 1862, elevating rest and relaxation to a top priority for enlisted men. Furloughs (never for more than sixty days) would be granted "to all twelve-months men now in service who shall, prior to the expiration of their present term of service, volunteer or enlist for the next two ensuing . . . or for three years, or the war. Said furloughs to be issued at such times and in such numbers as the Secretary of War may deem most compatible with the public interest, the length of each furlough being regulated with reference to the distance of each volunteer from his home." Transportation to and from furloughs would even be funded by the government. As soon as General Johnston heard the order, he feared the dissolution of his army. He wrote back to Secretary of War Judah P. Benjamin, "The terms both of the law and of the order in question leave my mind in doubt as to the time at which any person re-enlisting has the right to expect a furlough." After all, the order stipulated that Benjamin himself would decide, at the very least undercutting Johnston's authority over his men. Johnston continued, "I beg leave to submit for the consideration of the Department the impracticability of granting [furloughs] within the time specified in such numbers as will induce any considerable re-enlistments among the twelve-months regiments in this command, for the army here is composed in large part of such regiments, and inasmuch as the terms of service of nearly all of them expire at no distant day, it would be necessary to grant furloughs in very great numbers during the next few months, in order to obtain many re-enlistments for the two years following." Johnston knew a campaign was imminent and feared the ramifications of awarding leaves en masse. "To grant them in such numbers I deem incompatible with the safety of this command. The men here now are as few as we can safely meet the enemy with; yet there is no saying how soon he may attack us."[79]

The debate devolved into a power contest between Benjamin and Johnston. Benjamin replied, "I am aware that your solicitude for the safety of your command must necessarily embarrass you in giving furloughs in large numbers at present; but at the same time I beg you to observe that the eager desire for a furlough during the inclement season will form the strongest inducement for your men, and thus afford the best guarantee of your having under your orders a large force of veteran troops when active operations recommence." The secretary accordingly acknowledged that the worse the weather, the more men needed a break from soldiering. Veterans could be enticed to return if given this concession when environmental conditions were most grueling and active campaign least likely. Further, Benjamin implied that if the soldiers were not given the opportunity to recover now, they would straggle at an inopportune moment, such as in the middle of a campaign. "It seems scarcely possible that in the present condition of the roads an attack can be make; and it is surely better to run a little risk now than to meet the certain danger of finding a large body of your men abandoning you at the expiration of their terms, now nearly about to expire."[80] On this point, Benjamin would prove correct.

Johnston remained stingy with furloughs, despite the secretary of war's strong case in their favor. A month later, when he was called upon to send troops to aid Jackson in the Valley, Johnston reminded Benjamin of his original objections to the furlough system: "The reduction of our force by the operation of the furlough system makes it impracticable to re-enforce the Valley District from that of the Potomac." Several days later he reiterated the complaint: "The army is so much weakened by loss of officers from sickness and soldiers on furlough, that I am compelled to use every man in the way in which he can serve best."[81] The debate over furloughs had become an excuse rather than a serious discussion about army health.

As shown through this winter exchange, Benjamin took the longer view, realizing that winter furloughs produced more able-bodied, cheerful men who might reenlist. Johnston, typical of commanders in the field, saw that in the short term his army would be dangerously weakened and exposed. Lee, in the midst of his furor over deserters in the fall of 1862, revealed that he agreed with Johnston, going so far as to suggest that those on furlough should not receive pay, much like stragglers. He wrote to Secretary of War Randolph, "I have the honor to suggest, as one of the means of keeping men and officers with the army, that those who are absent on furlough or leaves of absence be not allowed to draw their pay while so absent." He believed such a policy would "hasten . . . their return, besides being more just to those who remain with the army."[82] Lee's subtle message was that the furlough was a practice that hurt rather than helped the cause.

Unsurprisingly, medical directors tended to side with army commanders on the issue of furloughs. For instance, Lafayette Guild, the Army of Northern Virginia's medical director, complained that those on leave suffered from more sickness than those retained and treated by the Medical Department. He argued that men who sought care outside of the army system did not receive sufficient medical treatment.[83] This indictment of home care served to reassert the primacy of the Medical Department in army health care. The soldiers' preference for civilian care was a challenge to army medical authority and a challenge to professional medicine as a whole, which had already been severely weakened in the Jacksonian era. Medical directors knew they would be blamed for sickly armies, and yet so many circumstances that shaped soldier health were beyond their control.

Conversely, regimental officers often fought for increased furloughs or, in lieu of official sanction, allowed men informal leave. Colonels witnessed firsthand their troops' weariness and sagging morale and understood that wintertime furloughs could keep their men loyal and healthy. The poor conditions experienced during the Romney campaign caused a number of regimental officers to voice their frustration over the lack of furloughs authorized by Stonewall Jackson. For instance, Col. Samuel V. Fulkerson wrote on January 23, 1862, to his Virginia congressman, Walter R. Staples, from Romney: "Now we are ordered to remain here during the remainder of the winter. A more unfavorable spot could not be selected. We are willing to endure all that men can bear when our cause requires it; but where there is a discretion, that discretion should be exercised in favor of men who have seen such hard and continued service." He continued, "We all must be impressed with the great importance of raising an army for the next summer. With the benefit of a short furlough for the men, I am satisfied that at Winchester I could have enlisted 500 of my regiment. . . . With the present prospect before them, I do not know that I could get a single man."[84] A group of General Loring's officers, Fulkerson included, included a plea for furloughs in their petition protesting the conditions at Romney. On January 25, 1862, they wrote: "The terrible exposure and suffering . . . can never be known to those who did not participate in it. When men pass night after night in the coldest period of a cold climate without tents, blankets, or even an ax to cut wood with, and without food for twenty-four hours," it was no wonder that an original force of 600 men when it left Winchester would be reduced to 200. Therefore, they suggested even a short furlough to revive men's spirits.[85] As historian Peter Carmichael explains, throughout the Romney and Valley campaigns Confederate regimental officers "astutely defused [class warfare] by granting informal 'French Furloughs,' a practice that allowed men to make brief trips home even though it violated military protocol at the most fundamental level." Carmichael confirms that this was particularly accepted "during winter quarters or lulls between campaigns."[86]

The Confederacy had a more severe manpower crisis than the Union in 1862, motivating this verbal contest over furloughs. Proof was in the culminating April 1862 draft. But the United States was hardly free from difficulty in filling the ranks. There was the occasional official discussion regarding overuse of furloughs. In July 1862, Maj. Gen. John E. Wool on the Virginia coast wrote to Secretary of War Stanton, "Measures ought to be adopted to apprehend and send back to their regiments the thousands of deserters scattered throughout the country. These with the men on furlough would make a respectable army."[87] Wool saw "desertion," by which he probably also meant straggling, and furloughs as comparable manpower problems. A similar situation existed in the Valley District. Assistant Secretary of War P. H. Watson wrote to Secretary Stanton, "The One hundred and second New York, which arrived this morning, had its colonel Hayward but neither lieutenant-colonel, major, quartermaster, nor commissary, these officers being on furlough. It would add greatly to the efficiency of our forces if every officer was at once ordered to join his regiment, unless unable to bear arms by reason of physical disability."[88] The persistent lack of officers attracted even President Lincoln's ire by November 1862. In a memo he lamented, "The Army is constantly depleted by company officers who give their men leave of absence in the very face of the enemy . . . which is almost as bad as desertion."[89] In these cases, regimental-level officers and common soldiers were being lumped into a similar category: volunteer soldiers who could not stand the rigors of soldiering and were shirking duty by taking leave.

To focus on the debate over furloughs appears to suggest that furloughs were frequently granted, when in fact enlisted men were largely deprived of leave during the active campaign season of 1862. As Private Pryor of Georgia explained from the Army of Northern Virginia, "It is verry hard for one to get off home from this command on sick furlough."[90] Thus, straggling became an essential component of self-care. On the one hand, it would have been destructive for military command to condone straggling, an overt breakdown of military discipline, but on the other, command could have better assessed the reasons for straggling and considered the furlough as a potential solution.[91]

Enlisted men, nevertheless, fully comprehended the significance of the furlough to their health. When Virginian Charles Elisha Taylor was sick, he longed for a proper leave. He had, in fact, just returned to his unit from convalescence in a civilian home, apparently too soon. He wrote to a friend, John. H. Horsham, for help. But Horsham responded, "I went to see Dr. Coleman as you requested and stated the facts to him, but he thought it was not necessary for you to have a furlough, I am sorry I could not succeed in procuring it for you." So Taylor continued to ail, his spirits plunging dangerously.[92] Such men fell through the cracks in 1862.

By the fall and winter of 1862, soldiers realized that straggling had become riskier business than it had once been. They had seen commanders misconstrue soldier motivations for quitting the ranks, and they had encountered civilian chastisements in the newspapers. While straggling would by no means end, the stakes of leaving the ranks to accomplish self-care had been raised. But junior officers would also remain allies of their men, protecting them from the uncompromising military goals of their commanders. Further, there was evidence that some of the reasons for straggling were being addressed; the logistical capacities and Medical Departments of the Confederacy and United States saw major advancements by year's end. But it is important to remember that just because both sides improved supplies, hospital access, and evacuation procedures does not mean the men grew more inclined to seek professional care. Many of the reasons to straggle for self-care remained as valid as ever, such as seeking private nursing, potable water, or a night away from the unremitting environmental hardships of soldiering.[93]

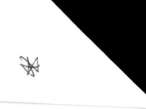

Self-Care beyond 1862

On May 22, 1862, New York artillerist George Perkins lay in camp listening to the thuds of hail "as big as marbles and some as big as English walnuts." Though his "little tent stood the storm well," the private was sodden and, over the course of the night, developed a raging fever. The next morning, he dropped out of his battery to wander the bewildering, washed-out roads of the Virginia Peninsula. That evening he fell in with some Michiganites, who took refuge in a barn. All night they heard rats scampering across the planks, stealing kernels of corn. A few days later, still sick and now itching with a mysterious rash, Perkins was back with his battery, a shade of his former self. On May 27, he scribbled in his diary, "Rained all last night and part of the day. . . . Sick with no care." On May 29, "Cloudy and rainy. Sick all the time." And finally, on June 4, "Drizzly and rainy all day. Longed very much for home."[1] The rain, the marching, and the physical pain of soldiering had grown almost unbearable.

Perkins's diary was echoed by hundreds of thousands of men in 1862 Virginia, most of whom saw relatively little of the horror and exhilaration of combat that year. They all, however, became fast experts in enduring the environmental misery of soldiering. Like Perkins, many of the men attempted to fasten their tents against exposure, intervene in their camp terrain, gather food and fresh water, straggle for reprieve, or practice other self-care techniques. They banded together in camp or on the march, or slipped quietly into barns, churches, or private homes, hoping to avoid the unfamiliar and inadequate army medical systems. The majority of the men still succumbed to illness or melancholy at some point during 1862, but actively adapting to their environments at least gave them a fighting chance to stay alive and mentally resilient.

On the one hand, self-care's emphasis on disease prevention, and its attention to boiling water, eradicating insects, and tempering exposure to filth anticipated a percolating medical revolution that would culminate in germ theory and vector-borne illness theory in the 1870s and 1880s. On the other hand, many of these folk cures and practices had been popular with the lower classes for decades, some even millennia. It was, however, the Civil War that provided the opportunity for average Americans to proliferate knowledge about health and nature and innovate with an unprecedented urgency. As the soldiers became seasoned to the environment of war, they surpassed those at home in the complexity of their understandings of how nature interacted with their bodies and mental states. It remains to be seen if this divergence changed the way veterans reintegrated into society and accepted or rejected postwar developments in environmental management, science, and medicine. Yet some aspects of self-care resulted in immediate estrangement between soldiers and their commanding officers and also between soldiers and civilians. The democratic spirit underlying self-care would only be tolerated to the degree that it did not appear to interfere with military operations and the progress of campaigns. Soldiers in 1862 exceeded those limits, drawing ridicule for their straggling, their indulgence in non-regulation food and supplies, and their apparent disregard for or perhaps ignorance of army protocols. To some, common soldiers appeared to have failed to adapt to military life. But from their own perspectives, the men had weathered immense challenges unfathomable to and often unacknowledged by outsiders. The soldier community encouraged and celebrated each other's self-care accomplishments as rungs on the ladder to coveted veteran status.

The process by which Confederates and Federals adapted to their environments in 1862 had proved remarkably similar. While Virginians occasionally navigated a different set of circumstances in that they were close to home and could straggle more easily to their families, all soldiers perceived and adapted to diverse environments in essentially identical ways. The question is to what extent the similarities between troops had to do with the year of the case study, before army infrastructures were fully developed and both sides were still struggling to support their armies in the field. In 1862 and beyond, the Union developed the more complex medical bureaucracy than the Confederacy, involving the U.S. Sanitary Commission and Jonathan Letterman's efficient system of ambulance evacuation, and enjoyed a more robust reserve of supplies, especially chemically manufactured medicines.[2] Further, the United States constructed more centralized and efficient methods for mobilizing citizens at home to support soldier health in the field, again largely thanks to Sanitary Commission.[3] While these advantages could be viewed as generating a reduced need for Union soldier self-care as the war proceeded, it is important to remember that the United States was also operating in hostile territory. This reality necessitated relying upon better evacuation, employing supplementary civilian hospital care at the home front, and protecting and operating extensive, vulnerable supply lines. Meanwhile the Rebel system, after being overwhelmed with sick and wounded during the Peninsula campaign, developed its own sophisticated hospital network that in Virginia alone included large complexes at such important hubs as Richmond, Petersburg, Gordonsville, Charlottesville, Lynchburg, and Danville, all connected by railroad.

In short, both sides established improved infrastructural support for soldiers after 1862. But to imagine that self-care was only necessary when supplies or rations were sparse and hospital availability was lacking would be to miss the point. Shortages did increase vulnerability, but even sleeping in a Sibley tent with a belly full of vegetables did not protect against the worst environmental dangers; diseases such as typhoid fever, diarrhea, and malaria still lurked in water sources, soil, and insect carriers. Soldiers would continue to avoid environmental circumstances they viewed as threatening or uncomfortable. Further, even with the best of equipment, five days of hard marching in the rain could spoil the most cheerful soldier's spirits if he did not actively fortify himself against mental decline. Union and Confederate soldier self-care therefore remained similar and indispensable even after 1862 because of shared cultural ideas about nature and disease causation and mutual preferences for self-reliance and privatized, familial care.

Thus, while this study continues a trend in common soldier scholarship of emphasizing soldier similarities and their material concerns in everyday life, it also moves beyond previous literature to offer new insights.[4] Not only did understanding and mitigating environmental impacts upon mental and physical health constitute soldiers' primary preoccupations outside of combat, but self-care prompted a great deal of the straggling in 1862 that historians have long recognized as problematic. While this narrative has privileged the soldier perspective, it is also easy to comprehend the frustration of military leaders with absenteeism. Straggling made waging campaigns an arduous task, and considering the great pressure generals were under from the governments and civilian populaces to deliver battlefield victories, it is not surprising that generals attacked straggling with more vigor than the seemingly impenetrable problems of disease,

vironmental management. While Civil War scholarship is
g-term study of straggling as distinct from desertion, the
ook suggest that strategic straggling was, in fact, healthy
volunteer units despite commanders' well-founded dis-
he practice.

᷒ historians can plainly benefit from employing the techniques
of environmental history, but environmental scholars should also consider
why a partnership with military history is vital to tracking the evolution
of American ideas about nature. Soldiers more than any other Americans
living in the nineteenth century developed a profound intimacy with their
environments. But even civilians and medical experts began to ponder
the novel wartime relationship between soldier bodies and nature. For
instance, on April 16, 1862, a piece authored by the Sanitary Commission
for the *Chicago Tribune* contemplated the decline of humoral theory in
favor of environmental explanations for disease. It posited that "interesting questions of inquiry in the science of 'Medical Topography' will grow
out of the experiences of the war, and will challenge the attention and
study of the Galens of the land."[5]

In a similar vein, and of particular interest to historians of science and
medicine, some physicians appeared to be affected by their observations
of soldiers interacting with nature. In a postwar publication prepared for
the Sanitary Commission, Dr. Batholow, a physician at the Medical College of Ohio and formerly a Civil War assistant surgeon, reflected that "the
recruit makes a sudden transition from a natural state to an artificial state
without any preparation for the change." The moment a soldier entered
the service, he was "hurried to the depot . . . supplied with army rations
badly cooked and uncleanly served; he is drilled vigorously . . . [given]
slender opportunities of washing and bathing," bombarded by the "unwholesome airs" of camp, and given insufficient cover for sleeping. "The
great change in his habits and modes of life, associated with so much that
was disagreeable and repulsive, induced in the recruit, if not possessed
of considerable fortitude and personal resources, a state of deep dejec-
tion, hypochondria, and nostalgia."[6] Batholow therefore connected the
environmental experience of soldiering to mental health, though he did
proceed to then privilege constitutional and racial explanations for disease
over environmental causes. In this way did certain soldiers' experiences
fold into the larger intellectual narratives taking place at mid-century.

Although soldiers attempted to establish continuity with their prewar
health experience and in many ways succeeded, the Civil War also became a special moment of transition. Because of the sheer size of Civil

War armies, never before had so many average men been forced to become creatures of the outdoors, so dependent on environmental adaptation for survival. For the first time, a staggering proportion of people suffered from illness and melancholy away from their homes and families and were forced to rely upon themselves, each other, or the emerging class of professionals. While diaries and letters reveal soldiers' struggles at the time with this foreign experience, their memoirs in the final decades of the nineteenth century betrayed a persistent longing to understand and interpret their wartime experiences with health and environment. In particular, veterans recast their epic confrontations with insects to reflect new knowledge that mosquitoes and flies transmitted disease.[7]

Despite soldiers' enduring fascination with the environment of war, historians have overlooked self-care because soldiers' interactions with nature appeared so banal. But environment was not static and the soldiers were not passive. Though the process of industrialization, which would alienate Americans from nature, barreled forward to support war mobilization, the soldiers themselves developed an almost primitive relationship with environment from the moment they left home for first camp. Dr. Batholow was astute when he called this transition to army life "artificial." There was nothing natural about the environment of war—a grotesquely human creation. But volunteer soldiers proved remarkably resilient, creating circumstances that fostered their own best chances for surviving the Civil War.

Figures

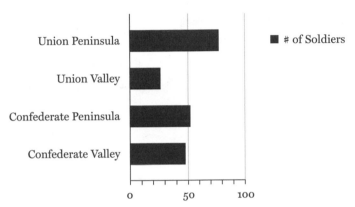

Figure 1. Number of soldiers sampled, by side and location

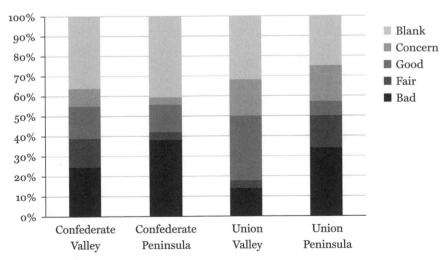

Figure 2. Soldiers' self-reported physical health as percentage of total, by side and location

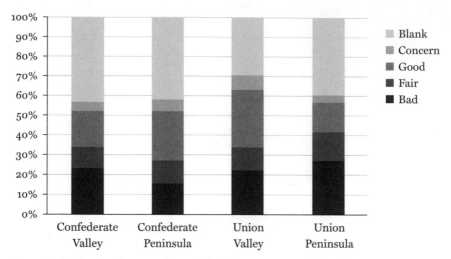

Figure 3. Soldiers' self-reported mental health as percentage of total, by side and location

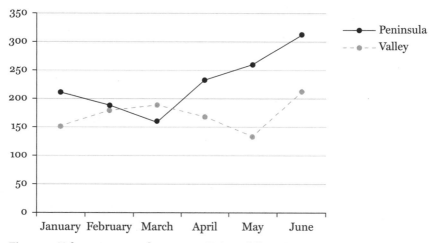

Figure 4. Sick cases reported per 1,000 Union soldiers, January–June 1862 (as recorded in *The Medical and Surgical History of the War of the Rebellion*, vol. 1, pt. 1)

Tables

Table 1. Overall Distribution of Self-Reported Health

COUNTRY, LOCATION, AND HEALTH	GOOD	FAIR	BAD	CONCERN FOR REGIMENT	BLANK	TOTAL
Confederate Peninsula, physical	7	2	20	2	21	52
Confederate Peninsula, mental	13	6	8	3	22	52
Confederate Valley, physical	8	7	12	4	18	49
Confederate Valley, mental	9	5	11	2	21	48
Union Peninsula, physical	6	13	27	14	20	80
Union Peninsula, mental	12	11	21	3	31	78
Union Valley, physical	9	1	4	5	9	28
Union Valley, mental	8	3	6	2	8	27
Total physical	30	23	63	25	68	209
Total mental	42	25	46	10	82	205

Note: The totals for location/health may be more than the number of soldiers in the sample because some soldiers were concerned about the health of their regiment in addition to expressing information about their own health.

Table 2. Correlations of Mental and Physical Health

(a) Confederate soldiers who reported on both mental and physical health (n=37)

	GOOD PHYSICAL HEALTH	POOR PHYSICAL HEALTH	FAIR PHYSICAL HEALTH
Good Mental Health	10	5	2
Poor Mental Health	0	10	0
Fair Mental Health	3	3	4

(b) Union soldiers who reported on both mental and physical health (n=47)

	GOOD PHYSICAL HEALTH	POOR PHYSICAL HEALTH	FAIR PHYSICAL HEALTH
Good Mental Health	10	2	3
Poor Mental Health	2	19	6
Fair Mental Health	1	4	0

Notes

BA   Boston Athenaeum Special Collections, Boston, Massachusetts

LVA   Library of Virginia, Archives and Manuscripts, Richmond, Virginia

MHS   Massachusetts Historical Society, Boston, Massachusetts

MOC   Eleanor S. Brockenbrough Library, Museum of the Confederacy, Richmond, Virginia

MSHWR   U.S. War Department, *The Medical and Surgical History of the War of the Rebellion: Prepared, in Accordance with the Acts of Congress, Under the Direction of Surgeon General Joseph K. Barnes, United States Army*, 6 vols., index and illustrations. Washington, D.C.: GPO, 1870–1888.

NYPL   New York Public Library, Humanities and Social Sciences, Manuscripts and Archives Division, New York, New York

OR   U.S. War Department, *The War of the Rebellion: A Compilation of the Official Records of the Union and Confederate Armies*, 129 vols., index and atlas. Washington, D.C.: GPO, 1880–1901.

USAMHI   Military History Institute, U.S. Army War College, Carlisle, Pennsylvania

UVA   Albert and Shirley Small Special Collections Library, University of Virginia, Charlottesville, Virginia

VSVCDH   "Valley of the Shadow: Two Communities in the American Civil War," Virginia Center for Digital History, University of Virginia, http://valley. VSVCDH.virginia.edu

INTRODUCTION

1. Pvt. Allen Seymour Davis, 1st Minnesota Infantry, to Charlie Davis, July 27, 1862, A. S. Davis Civil War Letters, UVA. Original spelling and grammar are preserved in all quoted soldier accounts.

2. According to James M. McPherson, "More than 90 percent of white Union soldiers and more than 80 percent of Confederate soldiers were literate, and most of them wrote frequent letters to families and friends" (McPherson, *For Cause and Comrades*, 11).

3. For instance, Anderson, *A People's Army*, and Winders, *Mr. Polk's Army*, capably prove that volunteer soldiers were sicker than regular soldiers in the Seven Years War and Mexican-American War, respectively.

4. Though it should be noted that not all army regulations were detailed enough to assist volunteer officers in their inexperience. Take, for instance, the regulations that

set parameters for protecting health in bivouac. "Reconnaissances should precede the establishment of the camp. For a camp of troops on the march, it is only necessary to look to the health and comfort of the troops, the facility of the communications, the convenience of wood and water, and the resources in previsions and forage"; in other words, there were no specifics delineating how "health and comfort" might be achieved (U. S. War Department, *Revised Regulations*, 74).

5. United States Sanitary Commission, Camp Inspection Report, 87th New York Infantry, January 1862, Series 1 Medical Committee Archives, 1861–65, and Series 7 Statistical Bureau Archives, Camp Inspection Reports, 1861–64, NYPL.

6. Harsh, *Taken at the Flood*; Carmichael, "So Far from God," and Bohannon, "Dirty, Ragged, and Ill-Provided For," are the best explorations of straggling as distinct from desertion. Works that tend to look at desertion and straggling as facets of the same problem include Weitz, *More Damning Than Slaughter*; Lonn, *Desertion during the Civil War*; Ruffner, "Civil War Desertion from a Black Belt Regiment"; Blair, *Virginia's Private War*; Glatthaar, *General Lee's Army*; Sheehan-Dean, *Why Confederates Fought*; Wetherington, *Plain Folk's Fight*; Cozzens, *Shenandoah 1862*; Reiger, "Deprivation, Disaffection, and Desertion in Confederate Florida."

7. As Pvt. Bailey George McClellan put it, "Food was no less a culprit of poor health and rampant disease. The Southern soldier was fed unsanitary, vermin-ridden food. Much of the sickness was caused by rancid beef" (McClellan, *I Saw the Elephant*, 16).

8. Billings, *Hardtack and Coffee*, 47–49.

9. The available statistics on disease remain notoriously unreliable, as the official Union records compiled in *The Medical and Surgical History of the War of the Rebellion* were muddled by misdiagnosis, underreporting, and failure to take note of the walking sick, while official Confederate records burned in the 1865 occupation of Richmond. Thus, only scattered regimental Confederate records remain. Statistics on morale are virtually non-existent, save the direst mental illnesses, such as nostalgia (potentially deadly homesickness), mania, insanity, or suicide. See, for instance, U.S. War Department, *MSHWR*, vol. 1, pt. 1:25–41, 174–80, and "Reports of Sick and Wounded, Taken sick or received into hospital" of Alabama, Virginia, and Georgia regiments, in Hunter Holmes McGuire Collection, oversize box 1, MOC.

10. This sample in this study is composed of 205 soldiers; see Figure 1 (Appendix 1). It should be noted that these percentages are relevant only to the sample. They cannot necessarily be extrapolated from to represent the whole of any given army. What the numbers do reflect is that many sick and depressed soldiers fell through the cracks of the official reporting system and the historical records. By studying individual accounts we can recover a health experience of common soldiers that is otherwise lost.

11. See Table 1 (Appendix 2) and Figures 2 and 3 (Appendix 1). The remaining soldiers did not provide enough information about their health to be conclusive and are referred to as "blank" in Table 1. Those men in "poor" health reported debilitating and persistent sickness, which means they suffered from a string of serious illnesses that either forced them into the hospital for long stretches or for repeated stints or incapacitated them from being able to complete their duties for large portions of the year. Men in "fair" health went to the hospital once or twice and/or suffered from more than one illness. Those deemed in "good" physical health either never reported illness

or suffered a very minor ailment, such as one sore throat or headache over the period of the sample. Those men deemed in "good" mental health remained cheerful throughout the duration of the two campaigns. Those with "poor" mental health consistently complained of attacks of "the blues," sadness, homesickness, and loneliness, and they wrote of refusing to leave their tents, rejecting duties, welcoming death, and/or feeling angry at their family members and situation. They also acted out in destructive ways, such as binge drinking or prompting disciplinary action. Those in "fair" mental health occasionally recorded intense feelings of sadness or homesickness but were able to recover.

12. Steiner, *Disease in the Civil War*, 12–13.

13. This is a type of seasoning covered extensively by Hess, *The Union Soldier in Battle*; but also investigated by Linderman, *Embattled Courage*; McPherson, *For Cause and Comrades*; and Mitchell, *Civil War Soldiers*.

14. The standard top-down studies of Civil War medicine are Steiner, *Disease in the Civil War*; Rutkow, *Bleeding Blue and Gray*; Adams, *Doctors in Blue*; Cunningham, *Doctors in Gray*; Green, *Chimborazo*; Freemon, *Gangrene and Glory*; Ashburn, *History of the Medical Department*; Schroeder-Lein, *Confederate Hospitals on the Move*; and Bollet, *Civil War Medicine*.

15. Downs writes that "tens of thousands of freed slaves became sick and died due to the unexpected problems caused by the exigencies of war and the massive dislocation triggered by emancipation" (Downs, *Sick from Freedom*, 7). In a somewhat similar vein, this book investigates how the circumstances of war and army movement, compounded by a lack of medical infrastructures, contributed to widespread sickness and death.

16. The standard works on the U.S. Sanitary Commission have tended to focus on the conflicts between the military and the Commission and between female and male leaders in the Commission, as woman sought to gain political footing. See Fredrickson, *The Inner Civil War*; Maxwell, *Lincoln's Fifth Wheel*; Giesberg, *Civil War Sisterhood*; Attie, *Patriotic Toil*; Greenbie, *Lincoln's Daughters of Mercy*; and Lori D. Ginzberg, *Women and the Work of Benevolence*. More in line with this book, Frances M. Clarke's *War Stories* investigates how the Sanitary Commission fostered the care of soldiers as individuals (Clarke, *War Stories*, 92).

17. See Batholow, "The Various Influences," 10–11, 15.

18. Several military scholars have incorporated environment into their narratives, but this is not their analytical focus; see Glatthaar, *General Lee's Army*; Cozzens, *Shenandoah 1862*; and Harsh, *Taken at the Flood*. Some historians of the common soldier have concentrated upon the material aspects of soldiering, most famously Wiley, *The Life of Johnny Reb* and *The Life of Billy Yank*; followed up by Glatthaar, *The March to the Sea and Beyond*; and then Mitchell, *Civil War Soldiers*. Works that have focused on the internal life of the soldier, including morale, are Linderman, *Embattled Courage*; Hess, *The Union Soldier in Battle*; and McPherson, *For Cause and Comrades*. And newer treatments of soldier ideology, religion, politics, and combat experience can be found in Barton and Logue, *The Civil War Soldier*; and Sheehan-Dean, *The View from the Ground*.

19. Clarke, *War Stories*, 10. Karen Lystra's earlier *Searching the Heart* did much the same.

20. See, most notably, Dean, "Dangled over Hell," 397; and Harsh, *Taken at the Flood*, 44–45.

21. Schantz, *Awaiting the Heavenly Country*, and Faust, *This Republic of Suffering*.

22. Valencius, *The Health of the Country*. Other environmental historians who have looked at the body in the nineteenth century include Stroud, "Reflections from Six Feet Under the Field"; Nash, "Finishing Nature"; and Brown, *Foul Bodies*.

23. The first two books to examine the Civil War from an environmental perspective are Brady, *War upon the Land*, and Nelson, *Ruin Nation*, preceded by a handful of articles and chapters, including Fiege, "Gettysburg and the Organic Nature of the Civil War"; Kirby, "The American Civil War"; Brady, "The Wilderness of War"; Taylor, "How a Cold Snap in Kentucky Led to Freedom for Thousands"; Meier, "Fighting in 'Dante's Inferno'"; and one chapter of Steinberg, *Down to Earth*, titled "The Great Food Fight," 89–98. Environmental histories of the nineteenth century that skipped over the war include Nash, *Wilderness and the American Mind*; Black, *Nature and the Environment in 19th-Century American Life*; and Cowdrey, *This Land, This South*.

24. While not employing the techniques of environmental history, there have been several military histories that have considered environment as formative aspects of the Civil War. See Winters et al., *Battling the Elements*, and Krick, *Civil War Weather in Virginia*.

25. This is not to say that certain diseases were not more prevalent in certain areas than others, but rather that all environments became dangerous to a degree in wartime. Andrew M. Bell has provided significant evidence that Arkansas was one of the unhealthiest places of the war—certainly more so than the Shenandoah Valley; however, this probably had more to do with the circumstances that heightened exposure (Bell, *Mosquito Soldiers*, 88–123).

26. See Figure 2 (Appendix 1), but note that the Union Valley sample is smaller than the other samples, slightly skewing those results. The Shenandoah Valley campaign concluded in early June, while the Peninsula campaign did not end until mid-August.

27. See Figure 4 (Appendix 1).

28. Of course, new recruits continued to be added to the ranks throughout 1862, bringing with them new waves of contagious disease. Further, it is important to note a disease like scurvy takes at least three months of vitamin C deprivation to set in, making 1862 the better year to investigate its effects.

29. Keith Bohannon discusses Confederate logistical improvements after the Antietam campaign, including a series of general orders improving the requisitioning of clothing, increased Quartermaster Department control of local supplies, and a reorganization of purchasing arrangements in the Commissary Department (Bohannon, "Dirty, Ragged, and Ill-Provided For," 130–31). George Rable similarly demonstrates improvements in logistics for the Army of the Potomac, thanks to Herman Haupt's efforts in "moving military supplies quickly over the railroads" (Rable, *Fredericksburg! Fredericksburg!*, 64–65).

30. Wyatt-Brown, *Southern Honor*; Camp, *Closer to Freedom*; Berry, *All That Makes a Man*; and Clarke, *War Stories* maintain fundamental differences between Northerners and Southerners. In the literature specific to Civil War soldiers, Reid Mitchell has pointed out that older scholarship, including his own and that of Bell Irvin Wiley,

Gerald Linderman, and Randall Jimseron, emphasize commonalities between Union and Confederate troops, while Earl Hess, Chandra Manning, and James McPherson emphasize contrasts (see Mitchell, "Not the General but the Soldier," 86–89).

31. The chosen sample purposely represents both published documents and unpublished manuscript collections to recognize that while it remains important to uncover new voices, we have also overlooked popular environmental health in the most familiar of soldier accounts.

32. Generals and medical directors, however, are excluded from the main sample, though their accounts are used to describe the official military medical systems in chapter 3.

33. Cushman, *Bloody Promenade*, is strong on parsing the difference between eyewitness accounts and reminiscences.

34. Linderman, *Embattled Courage*, 10, explains the stigma of cowardice for Civil War soldiers.

35. Barbara Sicherman notes the problematic nature of the phrase "mental health," which "reflects our ignorance" but also avoids implications of illness and embraces appropriate ambiguities (Sicherman, *The Quest for Mental Health in America*, 1).

36. As historian James M. McPherson has termed it, "The real battle was with the enemy, and the principal factors that shaped morale grew out of that conflict. These factors included the hardships, hunger, danger, shortages, and the like that were part of a soldier's lot." The "like" that he discusses, under which we might include environmental strain and disease, did not necessarily correspond to combat but merely the daily experience of being a soldier (McPherson, *This Mighty Scourge*, 162). See also, Dean, "Dangled over Hell," 400, which begins by suggesting that "marching, rain, snow, damp, and mud clearly had a depressing effect on the spirits and health of the men in Civil War armies" and that "biological warfare," or disease, devastated morale. The more standard reading of combat-based morale can be found in Maslowski, "A Study of Morale in Civil War Soldiers."

37. See Table 2 (Appendix 2).

38. The Union decision, historian Paul Steiner discusses, was made after a five-week study that showed that the Army of the Potomac would be almost destroyed by the Peninsula climate in August and September (Steiner, *Disease in The Civil War*, 142–43). On the Confederate side, in mid-August, Lee wrote to Jefferson Davis, "I think the health as well as discipline of the Army will be benefited by a change to the Country from the town & city itself receive a more healthy atmosphere" (Lee, *Lee's Dispatches*, 51).

39. Pryor, *A Post of Honor*, 150.

CHAPTER 1

1. Pvt. William R. Smith, 17th Virginia Infantry, diary [March 23 and 28, 1862, entries], Civil War Diary of William Randolph Smith, UVA.

2. James M. McPherson estimates that roughly fifty-six percent of Confederate enlisted men and fifty-two percent of Union enlisted men were farmers (McPherson, *For Cause and Comrades*, 181–82).

3. The tension between science and experiential knowledge was a common theme of the antebellum period, as evidenced by the public debate over whether book learning or experience was more important to farming practices; see Cohen, *Notes from the Ground*, 49–50.

4. Schantz, *Awaiting the Heavenly Country*, 10.

5. Common Americans did not avoid doctors when it came to surgery. Surgery had long been considered the domain of doctors, while care for illness had been much more diffuse. In addition, surgery had experienced a considerable advancement with the first demonstrations of anesthesia in the mid-1840s, beginning in dentistry (Rutkow, *Bleeding Blue and Gray*, 61; Rutkow, "Anesthesia during the Civil War," 680).

6. Valencius, *The Health of the Country*, 24.

7. Drake, "Selected Papers: Medical Topography," 137.

8. Cassidy, "Medical Men and the Ecology of the Old South," 166–79, 171.

9. See Nash, *Wilderness and the American Mind*, 23–43.

10. Patterson, "Disease Environments of the Antebellum South," 152; Warner, "The Idea of Southern Medical Distinctiveness," 179, 181; and Warner, "Public Health in the Old South," 226.

11. Hippocrates, *On Water, Airs, and Places*.

12. Brown, *Foul Bodies*, 303.

13. Bell, *Mosquito Soldiers*, 2.

14. Ibid., 12–13; Humphreys, *Intensely Human*, 45.

15. Webb, *Humanity's Burden*, 1–6; Patterson, "Disease Environments," 161. The final malarial strains—malarie and ovale—had limited to no influence upon the New World. American malarie was quite rare, while ovale probably did not extend beyond the African continent. The former had a disease cycle of seventy-two hours and, like falciparum, could be completely cured, while the latter recurred every forty-eight hours and lay dormant in its host, like vivax, recurring periodically.

16. Clarke, "Importance of Pure Air," *The Colored American*, August 15, 1840.

17. Schantz, *Awaiting the Heavenly Country*, 14–15.

18. "Traveling editorials," 469.

19. Lucas, "Observations on the Medical Topography and Endemic Fever of Montgomery County, Alabama," 78.

20. Somervail, "On the Medical Topography and Diseases of a Section of Virginia," 276.

21. Patterson, "Disease Environments," 162.

22. Thomson, "An Inquiry into the Medical Topography and Epidemic Fevers of the Valley of Virginia," 96.

23. Webb, *Humanity's Burden*, 9; Valencius, *Health of the Country*, 165–71.

24. Brown, *Foul Bodies*, 303, 230–31.

25. Schultz, *Women at the Front*, 20. Schultz expands that "in an era before its professionalization in the United States and well into the twentieth century, nursing was a manifestation of female identity and a domestic responsibility."

26. Valencius, *The Health of the Country*, 14.

27. Rosenberg, *The Care of Strangers*, 4.

28. Valencius, *The Health of the Country*, 54–55.

29. Brown, *Foul Bodies*, 213–14.

30. See Rosenberg, "Medical Text and Social Context," 22–42.

31. Buchan, *Domestic Medicine*, xii, 1.

32. Starr, *The Social Transformation of American Medicine*, 34.

33. Gunn, *Gunn's Domestic Medicine*, title page.

34. "The Water Cure Journal," *The National ERA*, June 24, 1852.

35. Clarke, "Importance of Pure Air," *The Colored American*, August 15, 1840.

36. Warner, *The Therapeutic Perspective*, 13–15.

37. Halliday, *The Great Filth*, 59.

38. See United States Sanitary Commission, *Report of a Committee . . . on the Subject of Scurvy*.

39. Lowry and Welsh, *Tarnished Scalpels*, xix, also provides a useful list of what every doctor presumably knew: to prescribe lime juice for the prevention and care of scurvy, to use quinine sulfate or Peruvian bark for malaria, to vaccinate against smallpox, to treat syphilis with mercury, and to control pain with opium. But not all "surgeons" in the Civil War were trained doctors.

40. Joseph Kett's *Formation of the American Medical Profession* provides an excellent summation of the descent of the medical field into sectarianism before the Civil War.

41. Warner, *The Therapeutic Perspective*, 24, 37.

42. Warner, "Orthodoxy and Otherness," 6.

43. Warner argues that this clinging to Hippocratic medicine served as a "recognizable badge of regular identity" (ibid., 10).

44. Valencius, *The Health of the Country*, 58–59, 54.

45. Rothstein, *American Physicians in the Nineteenth Century*, 42–45.

46. Whorton, *Nature Cures*, 6.

47. Warner, *The Therapeutic Perspective*, 98–99.

48. Kett, *The Formation of the American Medical Profession*, 155.

49. Haller, *American Medicine in Transition 1840–1910*, 18–20.

50. Ibid., 21.

51. Rosenberg, *No Other Gods*, 25, 27–28. Rosenberg notes that in the first quarter of the century, the mother was considered merely a receptacle for the father's seed; it was in the second quarter of the century that the mother's role in her offspring's development began to be scrutinized (30).

52. Ibid., 41–42.

53. Ray, *Mental Hygiene in America*, 12.

54. Mental health theories would have tremendous impact, however, on Civil War veterans after the war, a number of whom would be institutionalized based on wartime trauma (see McClurken, *Take Care of the Living*).

55. Rutkow, *Bleeding Blue and Gray*, 55–56, 59. See also Rutkow, "Homeopaths, Surgery, and the Civil War," 785–91.

56. Sicherman, *The Quest for Mental Health*, 4.

57. Barry, *The Great Influenza*, 25–27; Halliday, *The Great Filth*, 59, 79, 82–83.

58. Warner, "Orthodoxy and Otherness," 6; Rogers, *An Alternative Path*, 8. Historian Ira Rutkow suggests that alternative practitioners held at least equal footing in the court of public opinion (Rutkow, *Bleeding Blue and Gray*, 59).

59. Clarke, *War Stories*, 8–10.

60. Rogers, *An Alternative Path*, 4–5.

61. Barry, *The Great Influenza*, 7.

62. Rutkow, *Bleeding Blue and Gray*, 59.

63. Kett, *The Formation of the American Medical Profession*, 135–37.

64. "Botanico-Medical College of Ohio," *National ERA*, August 24, 1848.

65. Haller, *The History of American Homeopathy*, 247. For a contemporary source of information on Grahamism, see Campbell, *The Graham Journal of Health and Longevity*.

66. Rogers, *An Alternative Path*, 4–5.

67. Brown, *Foul Bodies*, 290–93, 308, 316.

68. Ibid., 200, 206, 290.

69. Halliday, *The Great Filth*, 23; Platt, *Shock Cities*, 141–44.

70. Brown, *Dorothea Dix*, 143.

CHAPTER 2

1. Capt. George Clark, 11th Alabama, *A Glance Backward: Or Some Events in the Past History of my Life* (1914; reprint, Ann Arbor: University Microfilms, 1973), USAMHI.

2. Haydon, *For Country, Cause & Leader*, 206.

3. Pvt. Lewis H. Bedingfield, 6th Georgia Infantry, to Pa and Ma, July 8, 1861, Bedingfield Family Civil War Letters, UVA. Sgt. Shepard G. Pryor wrote something very similar about his brother William in April 1862: "I got three letters from William. . . . I hope heel be able to stand it this time, for I dont want him here sick: it is the poorest place for a sick man I ever saw" (Pryor, *A Post of Honor*, 165). See also Pvt. Alan L. Bevan, 1st Pennsylvania Reserve Calvary, to parents, July 31, 1862, Bevan, John H. and Allen L. "Picketing along the Rappahannock," ed. Andrew W. German, VA Country's CW 8: pp. 32–38 (7 photocopied pages), USAMHI.

4. Lt. John Y. Bedingfield, 6th Georgia Infantry, to Pa and Ma, July 1, 1862, Bedingfield Family Civil War Letters, UVA.

5. Cozzens, *Shenandoah 1862*, 20–22, 25.

6. Apperson, *Repairing the March of Mars*, 227; Strother, *A Virginia Yankee in the Civil War*, 6.

7. Pvt. John C. Ellis, 111th Pennsylvania Infantry, to sister, June 15, 1862, Ellis, John C.—HCWRTColl-Ellis-MarshallFamilyColl, USAMHI.

8. Cozzens, *Shenandoah 1862*, 8, 50–51; Allan, *Jackson in the Shenandoah Valley*, 14–15.

9. Cozzens, *Shenandoah 1862*, 67, 69, 95, 98–99; Allan, *Jackson in the Shenandoah Valley*, 18–32.

10. While Loring's troops were stationed at Romney, Jackson's Surg. Hunter McGuire reviewed the sick and accused them of malingering. As a result, the surgeon sent 1,000 men back to active duty. Thus, there was some controversy over the extent to which Loring's soldiers were unduly suffering. Loring's petition to be removed to Winchester, which went over Jackson's head straight to Richmond, caused a stir that involved President Jefferson Davis and Secretary of War Judah P. Benjamin.

Consequently, Jackson did temporarily tender his resignation but asked to have it withdrawn several days later. The dispute was resolved in Loring's favor, as his soldiers were ultimately ordered back to headquarters at Winchester (Robertson, *Stonewall Jackson*, 314–22).

11. Allan, *Jackson in the Shenandoah Valley*, 33; Cozzens, *Shenandoah 1862*, 115.

12. Allan, *Jackson in the Shenandoah Valley*, 53–55; Long, *The Civil War Day by Day*, 190, 156–57.

13. Though Frémont's army operated in the same area as Banks's, sometimes within a proximity of fifty miles, the two men reported to different superiors (Banks to McClellan and Frémont to the War Department) and did not cooperate or coordinate, heightening miscommunication and supply problems (Miller, "Such Men as Shields, Banks, and Frémont," 45, 49–51).

14. Grayson, "Military Advisor to Stanton and Lincoln," 2:75–76.

15. Gallagher, "Introduction," in *The Shenandoah Valley Campaign of 1862*, viii–xiv; Allan, *Jackson in the Shenandoah Valley*, 92–94.

16. Long, *The Civil War Day by Day*, 187, 208, 215, 224; Gallagher, "You Must Either Attack or Give up the Job, " 8–15.

17. "Sanitary Statistics of the Army," *Chicago Tribune*, April 16, 1862.

18. *OR*, ser. 1, vol. 12, 3:9.

19. The Museum of the Confederacy in Richmond houses a number of these regimental medical reports, morning and monthly, from 1862. Used for this project were the Alabama, Virginia, and Georgia 1862 regimental reports ("Reports of Sick and Wounded, Taken Sick or Received into Hospital," Oversize Box 1, Hunter Holmes McGuire Collection, MOC).

20. Averell, *Ten Years in the Saddle*, 355–56.

21. Krick, *Civil War Weather*, 51, 54.

22. Long, *The Civil War Day by Day*, 193, 207, 222.

23. Burton, *Extraordinary Circumstances*, 402–3.

24. Long, *The Civil War Day by Day*, 231–33. For a more detailed explanation of these events, see Gallagher, *The Richmond Campaign of 1862*.

25. Summarized from Krick, *Civil War Weather*, 43–80.

26. Woodward, *Chief Camp Diseases*, 127; *OR*, ser. 1, vol. 11, pt. 1:211.

27. Calcutt, *Richmond's Wartime Hospitals*, 25. Steiner admirably attempts to compare Confederate and Union rates of sickness on the Peninsula throughout chapter 5 (Steiner, *Disease in the Civil War*, 98–146).

28. Lee, *Lee's Dispatches*, 51.

29. McCarthy, *Detailed Minutiae of Soldier Life*, 46.

30. Pvt. George Q. French, 3rd Vermont Infantry, diary [February 1 and 4, 1862 entry], G. Q. French Diary, 1862 January–September, LVA.

31. See Figure 4 (Appendix 1).

32. Cpl. John Bevan, 1st Pennsylvania Cavalry, letter to parents, February 2, 1862, "Picketing along the Rappahannock," USAMHI.

33. Morgan, *Personal Reminiscences of the War*, 98.

34. Maj. Frank B. Jones, 2nd Regiment Stonewall Brigade Infantry, diary [March 28 and April 10, 1862, entries], Frank B. Jones Diary, March-June 1862, MOC.

35. Pvt. Frasier Rosenkrans, 44th New York Infantry, to parents, June 11, 1862, Enlisted Men's Letters, Civil War Miscellaneous Collection, USAMHI.

36. Strother, *A Virginia Yankee in the Civil War*. See also Musc. Lewis C. Shepard, 7th Massachusetts Infantry, diary [January 10, 16, and July 17, 1862, entries], Lewis C. Shepard Diary, MHS; Perkins, *Three Years a Soldier*, 48, 50; Dwight, *Life and Letters of Wilder Dwight*, 240–41; and Morse, *Letters Written during the Civil War*, 52–53.

37. Carter, *Four Brothers in Blue*, 50.

38. Comey, *A Legacy of Valor*, 45.

39. Post, *Soldiers' Letters*, 89.

40. Pvt. Irvin C. Fox, 9th and 152nd Indiana Infantry, diary [March 10, 1862, entry], Civil War Diary of Irwin C. Fox 9th and 152nd Indiana, UVA. See also Miller, *Bound to Be a Soldier*, 26, and Pvt. Philip A. Lantzy, 40th Pennsylvania Infantry, to parents, May 24, 1862, Lantzy, Philip A.—HCWRTColl (Enlisted man's letters, July 27, 1861–August 24, 1862), USAMHI.

41. Haydon, *For Country, Cause & Leader*, 233.

42. Kearney, *Letters from the Peninsula*, 52.

43. Langstroth to wife, March 17, 1862, Langstroth, Thomas—CWMiscColl, USAMHI.

44. McCarthy, *Detailed Minutiae*, 45.

45. Huffman, *Ups and Downs of a Confederate Soldier*, 52.

46. Stewart, *Camp, March and Battle-field*, 200.

47. Haydon, *For Country, Cause, & Leader*, 238. See also Unknown, 11th Massachusetts Infantry, to Jim, July 29, 1862, Civil War letters of 11th Massachusetts Soldier 1611, UVA.

48. Lusk, *War Letters of William Thompson Lusk*, 169.

49. Pryor, *A Post of Honor*, 139.

50. Carter, *Four Brothers in Blue*, 70.

51. Haydon, *For Country, Cause & Leader*, 214. See also Warfield, *Manassas to Appomattox*, 73, and Norton, *Army Letters*, 97.

52. Ladley, *Hearth and Knapsack*, 38.

53. McClellan, *Welcome the Hour of Conflict*, 127.

54. Post, *Soldiers' Letters*, 44.

55. Pvt. David Watson, 53rd Virginia Infantry, to Mother, January 9, 1862, Letters of David Watson, 1861–62, UVA.

56. "The War in Virginia—A Reconnaissance in a Laurel Brake," *Harper's Weekly*, January 18, 1862.

57. Pvt. William F. Brand, 5th Virginia Infantry, to Kate, January 10, 1862, Papers of William Francis Brand, 1856–1959, UVA.

58. Pvt. Robert T. Hubard, 3rd Virginia Infantry, Notebook of Robert Thurston Hubard, 1860–1866, no page numbers, UVA.

59. Castleman, *Diary of Alfred Lewis Castleman*, 125.

60. Pvt. John O'Farrell, Crenshaw's Battery Artillery, diary [June 4, 1862, entry], John O'Farrell Diary, MOC.

61. Twichell, *The Civil War Letters*, 87–88. See also Surg. James R. Boulware, diary [April 19, 1862, entry], James Richmond Boulware Diary, 1862–1863, LVA.

62. Clark, *A Glance Backward*, 21.

63. Carter, *Four Brothers*, 231.

64. Le Duc, *Recollections of a Civil War Quartermaster*, 90.

65. Carter, *Four Brothers*, 51. See also Pvt. Smith diary [April 26, 1862, entry], Civil War Diary of William Randolph Smith, UVA, and Giles, *Rags and Hope*, 100–101.

66. Craig, *Captain Samuel A. Craig's Memoirs*, 23, USAMHI.

67. Beall, *Memoir of John Yates Beall*, 228.

68. Brown, *Campbell Brown's Civil War*, 131.

69. Carter, *Four Brothers in Blue*, 229.

70. Twichell, *The Civil War Letters of Joseph Hopkins Twichell*, 135–36.

71. Huffman, *Ups and Downs of a Confederate Soldier*, 55.

72. Norton, *Oliver Wilcox Norton*, 97.

73. Sgt. Keiser, *Diary of Henry Keiser of Lykens*, typescript, 23, USAMHI.

74. Pvt. Charles C. Perkins, 1st Massachusetts Infantry, diary [April 27 and May 19, 1862, entries], Perkins, Charles C.—CWTIColl, USAMHI.

75. Pryor, *A Post of Honor*, 148.

76. Miller, *Bound to Be a Soldier*, 26.

77. Carpenter, *War Diary of Kinchen Jahu Carpenter*, 8. See also Carter, *Four Brothers*, 214–15.

78. Pvt. W. H. Bird, 13th Alabama Infantry, Pvt. William H. Bird Memoir, 2, USAMHI.

79. Twichell, *Civil War Letters*, 142.

80. Pvt. Andrew W. Gillet, 52nd Virginia Infantry, to John Carpenter Eakle, July 13, 1862, Box 8169-a, UVA.

81. Billings, *Hardtack and Coffee*, 80.

82. Fletcher, *Rebel Private*, 9–10.

83. Billings, *Hardtack and Coffee*, 80–81. See also Holmes, *Touched with Fire*, 53.

84. Carter, *Four Brothers*, 93.

85. Billings, *Hardtack and Coffee*, 82.

86. Alfred Jay Bollet is a physician and historian who has questioned the presence of ticks in Civil War camps (Bollet, "Rheumatic Diseases among Civil War Troops," 1201).

87. Haydon, *For Country, Cause & Leader*, 238, 245.

88. Stewart, *Camp, March and Battle-field*, 147.

89. Huffman, *Ups and Downs*, 55. See also Post, *Soldiers' Letters*, 42, in which a soldier relates how the mosquitoes' "music" disturbed his sleep.

90. Pvt. John Leavitt, 26th Virginia Infantry, June 23, 1862, Letter book of John Leavitt, 1861–1865, p. 43, UVA.

91. Stewart, *Camp, March and Battle-field*, 149.

92. Bellard, *Gone for a Soldier*, 111–12.

93. Dunaway, *Reminiscences of a Rebel*, 23.

94. Pvt. Leavitt, June 23, 1862, Letter book of John Leavitt, 1861–1865, p. 43, UVA; Davis to sister, August 1, 1862, A. S. Davis Civil War Letters, UVA.

95. Fletcher, *Rebel Private*, 32–33.

96. Stewart, *Camp, March and Battle-field*, 209–10.

97. Perkins, *Three Years a Soldier*, 47.

98. Capt. Eugene Blackford, 5th Alabama Infantry, diary [June 1, 1862, entry], Blackford, Eugene—LeighColl Book 33 (MAJ's letters, March 11, 1861–September 2, 1862, and January 25, 1863–August 23, 1864; Misc. documents), USAMHI.

99. Pvt. Thomas Landers, 16th Massachusetts Infantry, to father and mother, April 5, 1862, Landers, Thomas—CWMiscColl (Enlisted man's letters, April 5 and May 21, 1862), USAMHI.

100. Fitzpatrick, *Letters to Amanda*, 16.

101. Private Blackington to Hannah, April 15, 1862, Blackington, Lyman and Jacob—BlackingtonColl, USAMHI.

102. Ellis, *Leaves from the Diary of an Army Surgeon*, 136.

103. Indeed, the numbers reported here only reflect this small soldier sample of 205 men.

104. *MSHWR*, vol. 1, 1:24–29, 37–39.

105. Steiner, *Disease in the Civil War*, 10.

106. Calcutt, *Richmond's Wartime Hospitals*, 25.

107. *MSHWR*, vol. 1, 1:30–35,174–80.

108. Steiner, *Disease in the Civil War*, 105–8.

109. "Reports of Sick and Wounded," Hunter Holmes McGuire Collection, MOC.

110. The reasons for variation among the regiments are addressed in the next chapter; they had to do with such factors as officer oversight of sanitation, placement of the regiment in a particular terrain, and how many of the soldiers were veterans versus new recruits.

111. See Table 1 (Appendix 2) and Figure 2 (Appendix 1).

112. See Figure 4 (Appendix 1).

113. *MSHWR*, vol. 1, 1:27–29, 33–35, 39–41, 176–79.

114. "Reports of Sick and Wounded," Hunter Holmes McGuire Collection, MOC.

115. See Table 1 (Appendix 2) and Figure 3 (Appendix 1).

116. Fitzgerald to Miss Sarah Appleton, July 31, 1861, and July 16, 1862, Haven-Appleton-Cutter Papers, 1692–1972, MHS.

117. Castleman, *Diary of Alfred Lewis Castleman*, 149.

118. Lowry and Welsh, *Tarnished Scalpels*, 106–8. Allegations against Castleman included using army hay to feed his own horse (officers were to provide their own hay), using hospital food to feed himself (again, officers were to pay for their own food), forbidding the apothecary and hospital stewards to prescribe medications because of their presumed incompetence, accepting money from two soldiers whom he helped to secure discharges, and ordering the dismissal of a disastrous assistant surgeon. At Castleman's trial most of the allegations were unsubstantiated, and the charges that held appeared to be instances in which Castleman feared that his subordinates' ineptitude might harm the soldiers.

119. Pvt. Fred R. Laubach, 93rd Pennsylvania Infantry, diary [May 25, 1862, entry], Fred R. Laubach Co. H, 93rd Pennsylvania Diary, 1862–1865, USAMHI.

120. Capt. Edward R. Young, 1st Virginia Artillery, diary [January 5, 1862, entry], "Civil War Papers of Edward Rush Young: Captain, Mount Vernon Guard and Young's Battery, C.S.A.," typescript, LVA.

121. Gache, *A Frenchman, a Chaplain, a Rebel*, 96.

122. There were 13 recorded suicides in the Union armies during the Peninsula and Shenandoah Valley campaigns and 391 for the entire war. No such data is available for the Confederate armies (*MSHWR*, v01.1 1:29, 35; Long, *The Civil War Day by Day*, 710).

123. Everson, *Stories of Our Soldiers*, 2:145.

124. Olmsted and Behling, *Hospital Transports*, 70.

125. Strother, *A Virginia Yankee in the Civil War*, 26.

126. *OR*, ser. 1, vol. 12, 3:52.

CHAPTER 3

1. Historian Charles E. Rosenberg writes that the Civil War marked a turning point when science played an increasing role in the minds of Americans. Though this transformation did occur to some extent over the course of the war, namely because of the efforts of the U.S. Sanitary Commission, soldiers often resisted the practices of traditional army surgeons in 1862 (Rosenberg, *No Other Gods*, 12).

2. Fred Shannon describes the conflicts between enlisted Federals and Union officers, and Peter Carmichael does the same for Virginians, emphasizing that privates relied upon their junior officers to smooth over tensions between themselves and their superiors (Shannon, "The Life of the Common Soldier in the Union Army, 1861–1865," 93; Carmichael, *The Last Generation*, 14).

3. Stewart, *Camp, March and Battle-field*, 74.

4. Clarke, *War Stories*, 51.

5. Stewart, *Camp, March and Battle-field*, 74.

6. For instance, George M. Fredrickson wrote that the elite leaders of the U.S. Sanitary Commission "welcomed the sufferings and sacrifices of the hour because they served the cause of discipline in a broader sense than demanded by purely military requirements. An unruly society, devoted to individual freedom, might be in the process of learning that discipline and subordination were good in themselves, and the commissioners wanted to play their role in teaching this lesson" (Fredrickson, *The Inner Civil War*, 105).

7. Stewart, *Camp, March and Battle-field*, 74.

8. Pvt. Albert M. Liscom, 13th Massachusetts Infantry, May 23, 1862, Albert M. Liscom Letters, Box 58, USAMHI.

9. Carpenter, *War Diary of Kinchen Jahu Carpenter*, 9.

10. Castleman, *Diary of Alfred Lewis Castleman*, 116.

11. Eliza Newton Woolsey Howland to Joseph Howland, in Howland, *Letters of a Family*, 360.

12. This evolution is something Frances Clarke notes; further, the "USSC's message took on increased sentiment and religious overtones as war continued" (Clarke, *War Stories*, 92–93).

13. Pvt. Lewis C. Shepard, 7th Massachusetts Infantry, diary [June 4, 1862, entry], Lewis C. Shepard Diary, MHS.

14. Pvt. William H. Bird, 13th Alabama Infantry, Pvt. William H. Bird Memoir, 4, USAMHI.

15. Clarke explains, "Individuals responded to . . . suffering in class-specific ways. . . . And they shared class-based understandings of suffering, too, especially a belief that other classes and races were less prone to suffering and less capable of sympathizing with distress." Clarke, however, also writes that Northern voluntary workers, such as members of the Sanitary Commission, saw what they wanted to see in soldiers in the hospitals: exemplary sufferers (Clarke, *War Stories*, 9, 59).

16. Castleman, *Diary of Alfred Lewis Castleman*, 72–74.

17. Edmonds, *Memoirs of a Soldier, Nurse and Spy*, 28.

18. Potter, *Notes of Hospital Life*, 108.

19. McClellan, *I Saw the Elephant*, 17.

20. Pvt. George Q. French, 3rd Vermont Infantry, diary [May 28–29, 1862, entry], G. Q. French Diary, 1862 January-September, LVA.

21. Keiser, *Diary of Henry Keiser of Lykens*, typescript, 29, USAMHI.

22. Pvt. Irvin C. Fox, 9th and 152nd Indiana Infantry, diary [March 10, 11, and 24, 1862, entries], Civil War Diary of Irwin C. Fox 9th and 152nd Indiana, UVA.

23. Haydon, *For Country, Cause & Leader*, 213–14.

24. Pvt. Aaron E. Bachman memoir, 10, Bachman, Aaron E.–HCWRTColl, USAMHI.

25. Pvt. Oscar Bailey, 1st Massachusetts, to mother, August 10, 1861, Bailey Family Letters, 1842–1866, MHS.

26. Strother, *A Virginia Yankee in the Civil War*, 31.

27. Pryor, *A Post of Honor*, 135.

28. Gache, *A Frenchman, a Chaplain, a Rebel*, 109.

29. Frederick Newman Knapp diary [June 14, 1862, entry], Frederick Newman Knapp Papers, MHS.

30. Pvt. Ephraim A. Wood, 13th Massachusetts Infantry, diary [July 3, 1862, entry], Journal of Private Ephraim A. Wood, UVA.

31. Post, *Soldiers' Letters*, 44–45.

32. Twichell, *The Civil War Letters of Joseph Hopkins Twichell*, 141.

33. United States Sanitary Commission, "Hospital Directory Paper pertaining to the Final Report, 1866," U.S. Sanitary Commission Washington Hospital Directory Archives, Box 192.3, NYPL.

34. While the Confederacy did not have a parallel institution to the U.S. Sanitary Commission, it did possess individual ladies' aid societies, which did not have as much direct interaction with soldiers but received equal praise. See, for instance, the *Richmond Dispatch* of January 3, 1862, which praised the patriotic efforts of the "Ladies' Ridge Benevolent Society" for caring for the dependent families of soldiers at war and donating wool to make socks for the men. On June 6, 1862, it singled out the "Ladies' Soldiers' Aid Society for the Natural Bridge District," who had invited "one hundred of our wounded soldiers to make their houses their homes during their convalescence."

35. War Department, *Revised Regulations*, 74–75.

36. Ibid., 76. As historian Glenna Schroeder-Lein explains, in some of the camps latrine sanitation meant shoveling six inches of dirt over the waste every day. Sometimes officers would instruct the men to mix in a bit of carbonic acid or chlorinated lime as

sanitizer, but this was rare in 1862 Virginia (Schroeder-Lein, *The Encyclopedia of Civil War Medicine*, 177–78).

37. Historian Peter Cozzens, for instance, presents the contrast between Brig. Gen. Richard B. Garnett's care of the Stonewall Brigade, which helped keep sickness low, and Brig. Gen. William W. Loring, who did not attend to sanitation and therefore had very sickly men (Cozzens, *Shenandoah 1862*, 43–44, 90).

38. Cpl. Washington Hands, Confederate 1st Maryland Infantry, Washington Hands Civil War Notebook, 1886 (handwritten), 40, UVA.

39. McClellan, *Welcome the Hour of Conflict*, 127.

40. Schroeder-Lein, *Encyclopedia of Civil War Medicine*, 177–78.

41. Winders, *Mr. Polk's Army*, 145–51, estimates that disease rather than combat accounted for 80 percent of Mexican War casualties.

42. Adams, *Doctors in Blue*, 4–5, 8.

43. Ibid., 10–11.

44. Strong, *Origin, Struggles and Principles*, 3, 5–6.

45. For more on the split between WCAR and the Sanitary Commission, particularly in terms of gender, see Giesberg, *Civil War Sisterhood*, 31–50.

46. Stillé, *History of the U. S. Sanitary Commission*, 50, 60, 63.

47. United States Sanitary Commission, *Documents of the U.S. Sanitary Commission*, 1:4, 1.

48. Stillé, *History of the U. S. Sanitary Commission*, 84–88.

49. United States Sanitary Commission, *Documents of the U.S. Sanitary Commission*, 1:9–11, 15, 18.

50. Adams, *Doctors in Blue*, 13. McClellan directed his surgeons through General Order 51 on August 3, 1861, and General Order 104 on December 3, 1861.

51. Rutkow, *Bleeding Blue and Gray*, 99.

52. Stillé, *History of the U. S. Sanitary Commission*, 515.

53. United States Sanitary Commission, "Object of the Examination," 1862 pamphlet, untitled bound volume (S.l.: s.n., 1862), MHS. Other information collected was about constitution: "What size, form, and weight of men are best adapted to the different branches of the service, and the effect of each service upon the men" and "the dimensions and proportions of soldiers, for the attainment of knowledge respecting the proportions of the human race, since the most vigorous constitutions and the years of best development are to be found in the military service." Inspectors specifically noted soldiers' names; heights; the measurements of their arms, pelvis, and shoulders; facial features; marital status; muscle quality; teeth; athleticism; education; vision; etc.

54. Adams, *Doctors in Blue*, 29–36.

55. Hammond, "Circular No. 2," May 21, 1862, Circulars and Circular Letters from the Surgeon General's Office, 1862–1865, U.S. Sanitary Commission, N0.1077–1081, NYPL.

56. Dougherty, *Civil War Leadership and Mexican War Experience*, 27.

57. U. S. War Department, General Order 106, March 16, 1864, http://www.civilwarhome.com/congressambulanceact.htm.

58. Cunningham, *Doctors in Gray*, 106.

59. *Staunton Spectator*, April 15 and June 6, 1862, VSVCDH.

60. Schroeder-Lein, *Confederate Hospitals on the Move*, 97.

61. Cunningham, *Doctors in Gray*, 28–30, 36.

62. Olmsted, *The Papers of Frederick Law Olmsted*, 4:353, 369.

63. Henry Bellows to Mr. W. Van Buren, May 13, 1862, Henry Bellows Papers, MHS.

64. Taylor, "Some Experiences of a Confederate Surgeon," 105, 115.

65. *OR*, ser. 1, vol. 12, 1:6.

66. Ibid., 3:40–41, 63, 197; Cozzens, *Shenandoah 1862*, 385.

67. *OR*, ser. 1, vol. 12, 1:10.

68. *OR*, ser. 1, vol. 12, 1:25. Historian Peter Cozzens has identified that at least some of the Union logistical problems in the Valley had to do with the U.S. War Department diverting troops and supplies to the campaign deemed more important: the Peninsula campaign (Cozzens, *Shenandoah 1862*, 48, 384).

69. While Frémont's army was most critically deprived, the other two major U.S. armies in the Valley—those of Banks and Shields—were also suffering from lack of shoes, demoralization, and few defenses against the bitter spring weather. Like Frémont, these generals were not able to overcome logistical and environmental problems to support their soldiers' health (see *OR*, ser. 1, vol. 12, 3:334, 339, for Shields, and *OR*, ser. 1, vol. 12, 3:52; 1:532–34, and Charles Sumner, *The Selected Letters of Charles Sumner*, 2:116, for reports on Banks).

70. Suckley's most famous naturalist publication was Suckley, Cooper, et al., *The Natural History of Washington Territory*.

71. *OR*, ser. 1, vol. 12, 1:30–31.

72. *OR*, ser. 1, vol. 12, 3:683, 262.

73. Grayson, "Military Advisor to Stanton and Lincoln," 1:75–76.

74. As quoted from Brig. Gen. Alexander R. Lawton, who served under Jackson in the Valley, in Glatthaar, *General Lee's Army*, 135. Though Jackson had paused in January of 1862 to allow his men to attend to bathing and picking off the lice that had infested their filthy clothing, he refused furloughs and did not allow for such a pause again once the spring campaign commenced, lending credence to Lawton's words (Tanner, *Stonewall in the Valley*, 76).

75. Surgeon William Riddick Whitehead, 44th Virginia Infantry, "A 19th Century Memoir: Adventures if an American Surgeon," 1862, transcript Karen F. McComas and Frances B. Ross, 2002, no page numbers, UVA. It was not just Confederate surgeons who were denied the possibility of moving camp for health reasons; Union surgeon Alfred Castleman had a similar complaint in winter of 1862. Castleman recalled in January of 1862 how carelessly the men were left to suffer in the winter. "The time has passed to move. But why are we not ordered to winter quarters? There seems to me to be great recklessness of the soldiers' health and comfort in this army" (Castleman, *Diary of Alfred Lewis Castleman*, 79).

76. Cunningham, *Doctors in Gray*, 261, 114.

77. As Pvt. Marion H. Fitzpatrick, a soldier in the Army of Northern Virginia, described, "The hospitals are overflowing and there is no chance to get them in." He, like many, had to move his sick friend to a private residence (Fitzpatrick, *Letters to Amanda*, 7). See also Lt. John Y. Bedingfield to parents, July 1, 1862, Bedingfield Family Civil War Letters, UVA.

78. McClellan, *McClellan's Own Story*, 349.

79. Castleman, *Diary of Alfred Lewis Castleman*, 147.

80. Smith, *Swamp Doctor*, 25. Smith reported that more than twenty-five percent of his regiment was "dead of malaria or too sick to move" (13).

81. Steiner, *Disease in the Civil War*, 114–15; Welsh, *Medical Histories of Union Generals*, 209–10.

82. McClellan, *The Civil War Papers of George B. McClellan*, 290.

83. *OR*, ser. 1, vol. 11, 3:70, 358, vol. 12, 3:46.

84. McClellan, *Civil War Papers*, 450.

85. Miller, "I Wait Only for the River," 44–65.

86. Lowry and Welsh, *Tarnished Scalpels*, 176.

87. *OR*, ser. 1, vol. 11, 1:181.

88. *OR*, ser. 1, vol. 11, 3:228–29.

89. Small, *The Road to Richmond*, 197.

90. *OR*, ser. 1, vol. 11, 3:191. In contrast to Tripler's statement, see official Union sick estimates on the Peninsula in *OR* ser. 1, vol. 11, 1:211, and Woodward, *Chief Camp Diseases*, 127.

91. Tripler wrote that "all sorts of doctors—steam, electric, and even advertising quacks—were sometimes commissioned as medical officers . . . men who had never even seen, much less performed, a surgical operation." In historian Paul Steiner's account of Peninsula health, he pardoned Tripler for spot-checking his numbers and for perceiving what we would now consider a dire health situation as simply par for the course in contemporary military reality (Steiner, *Disease in the Civil War*, 128).

92. Ashburn, *History of the Medical Department*, 72.

93. *OR*, ser. 1, vol. 11, 3:349.

94. See Dyer, *The Journal of a Civil War Surgeon*, 24–25.

95. *OR*, ser. 1, vol. 11, 3:350.

96. *OR*, ser. 1, vol. 11, 3:326–27.

97. *OR*, ser. 1, vol. 11, 1:215.

98. Steiner, *Disease in the Civil War*, 119, 139–40. Historian Paul Steiner makes much of the Confederate medical advantage over the Union on the Peninsula, while at the same time citing a rate of over twenty-five percent sick Confederates. He credits the Confederate army with avoiding scurvy in 1862, and while reports are spotty on this epidemic in the Army of Northern Virginia, July ledgers signaled the first appearance of consistent fruits and vegetables in the Confederate rations. Scurvy was the most likely impetus for this change. It takes at least three months or more for vitamin C deficiency to manifest as scurvy, and it makes sense that both Confederate and Union armies would have shown symptoms around the same time. (J. S. Melvin, Capt. and Adjutant Commissary of Subsistence, "The Subsistence Ledger 1862 Sept. 1–1863 July 31," Confederate States of America, 2nd Virginia, Stonewall Brigade, BA. The listed dates are a misnomer—the ledger actually covers 1861 through 1863.)

99. Welch, *A Confederate Surgeon's Letters to His Wife*, 60.

100. Bell, *Mosquito Soldiers*, 2; Webb, *Humanity's Burden*, 119.

101. Johnston had served as a topographical engineer in the Florida Seminole Wars, as an officer in key Mexican War actions, and, shortly before resigning his commission

during the secession crisis, as quartermaster general of the United States Army, eventually promoted to head of the Department of Northern Virginia (Symonds, *Joseph E. Johnston*, 43, 91, 150).

102. Johnston, *Narrative of Military Operations*, 65–66.

103. *OR*, ser. 1, vol. 11, 1:403–11, 66–67. Maj. Gen. John B. Magruder noted that Confederate command left health entirely up to the Medical Department. "The medical officers deserve the highest commendation for the skill and devotion with which they performed their duty in this sickly country" (*OR*, ser. 1, vol. 11, 1:403).

104. Glatthaar, "Confederate Soldiers in Virginia, 1861," 45–63.

105. Glatthaar, *General Lee's Army*, 145–46.

106. For an in-depth look at Lee's early leadership weaknesses see Harsh, *Taken at the Flood*.

107. Lee, *Lee's Dispatches*, 48, 51.

108. Cunningham, *Doctors in Gray*, 109–10, 113, 206.

109. See as examples United States Sanitary Commission, Camp Inspection Report 87th New York Infantry, January 1862; Camp Inspection Report 106 Pennsylvania Infantry, December 21, 1861; and Camp Inspection Report 53rd Pennsylvania Infantry, January 11, 1862, in Series 1 Medical Committee Archives, 1861–65, and Series 7 Statistical Bureau Archives, Camp Inspection Reports, 1861–64, United States Sanitary Commission Records, NYPL. Also see Stephen and McBride, "Civil War Housing Insights from Camp Nelson, Kentucky," 156.

110. Stillé, *History of the United States Sanitary Commission*, 99.

111. Olmsted and Behling, *Hospital Transports*, 60.

112. Twichell, *Civil War Letters*, 117–18.

113. Craighill, *Confederate Surgeon*, 40.

114. Castleman, *Diary of Alfred Lewis Castleman*, 162.

115. Monteiro, *War Reminiscences*, 21, 23.

116. Castleman, *Diary of Alfred Lewis Castleman*, 114, 157–58.

117. Dyer, *The Journal of a Civil War Surgeon*, 20.

118. Castleman, *Diary of Alfred Lewis Castleman*, 85, 91, 96.

119. Dyer, *The Journal of a Civil War Surgeon*, 17, 24–25.

120. Taylor, "Some Experiences of a Confederate Surgeon," 105, 115.

121. United States Sanitary Commission, *Report of a Committee . . . on the Subject of Continued Fevers*, 6–7, 16–17; Metcalfe, *Report . . . on the Subject of the Nature and Treatment of Miasmatic Fevers*, and Van Buren, *Report of a Committee . . . on the Use of Quinine*, 6.

122. We now understand that soldiers contracted diarrhea for a number of reasons — among them, amoebic, bacterial, protozoal, viral, helminthic, chemical, and metabolic (Steiner, *Disease in the Civil War*, 16–17).

123. United States Sanitary Commission, *Report of a Committee . . . on Dysentery*, 22–25; United States Sanitary Commission, *Report of a Committee . . . on Scurvy*, 16–25.

124. Wood, *Doctor to the Front*, 33.

125. Smith, *Swamp Doctor*, 25–27.

126. Dyer, *The Journal of a Civil War Surgeon*, 28.

127. Perry, *Letters from a Surgeon*, 18–19.

128. Smith, *Swamp Doctor*, 15. Surgeon Dyer also complained that one of his assistants "has been sick a week with remittent fever. I have a good deal to do and find it very tedious to spend four or five hours at surgeon's call." Just five days later, his assistant was still sick, as was the brigade surgeon. "I am well and attend to the business of both," wrote a weary Dyer, who was stretched too thin to provide adequate care (Dyer, *The Journal of a Civil War Surgeon*, 25–26).

129. Castleman, *Diary of Alfred Lewis Castleman*, 75, 98–99.

130. Ibid., 154–55.

131. *Valley Spirit*, February 19, 1862, VSVCDH.

132. Fletcher, *Rebel Private*, 13, 34. Fletcher related the story: "So one morning, while our mess was eating, I found what I supposed was a cat's claw and all stopped eating at once and an examination was hurriedly made of the uneaten portion, and a cat's tooth was discovered." Sure enough, "A report of the find was soon circulated and it was said that there were other finds of a similar character. Sausage was sold by weight and the more bone, the heavier."

133. *Valley Spirit*, February 19, 1862, VSVCDH.

134. "Sanitary Statistics of the Army," *Chicago Tribune*, April 16, 1862.

135. "The Health of the Army," *Christian Recorder*, December 28, 1861.

136. "Regimental and Brigade Hospitals," *Christian Recorder*, December 28, 1861; see also *Christian Banner*, June 18, 1862.

137. "The Army of the Potomac," *Harper's Weekly*, July 12, 1862.

138. "Regimental and Brigade Hospitals," *Christian Recorder*, December 28, 1861; see also "Increased Cost of Medical Attendance," *Richmond Daily Dispatch*, March 26, 1862, NYPL. See also "The General Hospital at Fortress Monroe," *Harper's Weekly*, June 7, 1862.

139. "General McClellan's Advance," *Harper's Weekly*, May 31, 1862; see also "The Sanitary Ship," *Harper's Weekly*, June 28, 1862.

CHAPTER 4

1. See Table 2 (Appendix 2).

2. McKim, *A Soldier's Recollections*, 84–85. McKim based his recollections on his diary.

3. Private Wood diary [July 5, 1862, entry], Journal of Private Ephraim A. Wood, UVA; for rough estimates of the weather in July see Krick, *Civil War Weather in Virginia*, 65. For other examples of bathing improving spirits, see Private Blackington diary [April–August 1862 entries], Blackington, Lyman and Jacob—BlackingtonColl, USAMHI, and Sgt. William H. West, 6th Maine Infantry, diary [April 18, 1862, entry], William H. West Papers, MHS.

4. Brown, *Foul Bodies*, 206.

5. As a general point of reference, *The Medical and Surgical History of the War of the Rebellion* reported roughly 1,159 cases of sunstroke on the Peninsula and in the Valley; most of these cases were on the Peninsula in July and August, during which temperatures soared into the mid-nineties. Overheating and dehydration took a significant toll on the soldiers' fitness for duty (*MSHWR*, vol. 1, 1:27, 33, 39, 175).

6. Lt. Jacob W. Haas, 96th Pennsylvania Infantry, diary [May 2, 1862, entry], Haas, Jacob W.—HCWRTColl, USAMHI. See also Lt. Valentine W. Southall, 23rd Virginia Infantry, to parents, June 14, 1862, Southall, V.W.—HCWRTColl-GACColl, USAMHI, who noted hundreds of bathers in his vicinity after a fatiguing march.

7. Patterson, *Yankee Rebel*, 36.

8. Howe, *Journals and Letters*, 491.

9. Corporal Hands, Washington Hands Civil War Notebook, 40, UVA.

10. Sergeant West diary [February 6, 1862, entry], William H. West Papers, MHS.

11. Howe, *Journals and Letters*, 491.

12. Pvt. Thomas M. Smiley, 5th Virginia Infantry, diary [July 25, 1862, entry], VSVCDH.

13. Private Smith diary [March 28, 1862, entry], Civil War Diary of William Randolph Smith, UVA.

14. Cpl. John Bevan to parents, April 3, 1862, "Picketing along the Rappahannock," USAMHI.

15. Stilwell, *The Stilwell Letters*, 10.

16. Haydon, *For Country, Cause & Leader*, 242.

17. Billings, *Hardtack and Coffee*, 85.

18. Langstroth to wife, May 2, 1862, Langstroth, Thomas—CWMiscColl, USAMHI.

19. Pvt. James P. Williams, 1st Pennsylvania Cavalry, to Nannie, June 17, 1862, Papers of James Peter Williams 1854–1889, UVA.

20. McClellan, *Welcome the Hour of Conflict*, 125. See also Hite, *The Painful News I Have to Write*, 75.

21. Pvt. Alvin N. Brackett, 1st Maine Calvary, to parents, June 11, 1862, Brackett, Alvin N.—HCWRTColl-GACColl, USAMHI.

22. Shepard diary [January 6, 1862, entry], Lewis C. Shepard Diary, MHS.

23. Blackington to sister, June 10, 1862, Blackington, Lyman and Jacob—BlackingtonColl, USAMHI.

24. Pvt. C. Perkins diary [April 11, 1862, entry], Perkins, Charles C.—CWTIColl, USAMHI.

25. McClellan, *Welcome the Hour of Conflict*, 128.

26. Brown, *Campbell Brown's Civil War*, 113.

27. Historian Megan Kate Nelson has demonstrated that encampments decimated forests (Nelson, *Ruin Nation*, 116–20).

28. Capt. Edward R. Young, 1st Virginia Artillery, diary [May 5, 1862, entry], "Civil War Papers of Edward Rush Young: Captain, Mount Vernon Guard and Young's Battery, C.S.A.," typescript, LVA.

29. Pvt. C. Perkins diary [June 7, 1862, entry], Perkins, Charles C.—CWTIColl, USAMHI.

30. Private Billings describes the various tents and their uses in *Hardtack and Coffee*, 47–49.

31. Major Jones diary [March 15 and April 18 and 21, 1862, entries], Frank B. Jones Diary, March-June 1862, MOC.

32. Castleman, *Diary of Alfred Lewis Castleman*, 98–99.

33. Everson, *Stories of our Soldiers*, 2:89.

34. "Building Huts for the Army of the Potomac," *Harpers' Weekly*, January 18, 1862.

35. Everson, *Stories of our Soldiers*, 2:89–90.

36. Hubard, Notebook of Robert Thurston Hubard, 1860–1866, no page numbers, UVA.

37. Post, *Soldiers' Letters*, 81.

38. Cpl. Joseph E. Blake, 12th Massachusetts Infantry, to parents, July 9, 1862, Blake, Joseph E.—CWMiscColl, USAMHI.

39. Haydon, *For Country, Cause & Leader*, 265.

40. Watson to mother, February 19, 1862, Letters of David Watson 1861–62, UVA.

41. Fletcher, *Rebel Private*, 16.

42. Pvt. Aaron E. Bachman, 1st Pennsylvania Cavalry, memoir, 9, Bachman, Aaron E.—HCWRTColl (Enlisted man and prisoner of war's memoirs, July 1861–July 1865), USAMHI.

43. Pvt. Lorenzo N. Pratt, 1st New York Light Artillery, to father, April 10, 1862, Pratt, Lorenzo N.—CWMiscColl (Enlisted man's letters, November 1861–December 26, 1864; Discharge & news article), USAMHI. The aforementioned Yorktown soldier also described "sassafras bushes, the roots of which are pleasant to eat, and are therefore pulled up without regard to quantity" (Post, *Soldiers' Letters*, 81).

44. Bellard, *Gone for a Soldier*, 111–12.

45. As explained earlier, draining one's camp also helped prevent mosquito eggs from hatching near the tents (Watson to mother, February 19, 1862, Letters of David Watson 1861–62, UVA). Very rarely, soldiers would mention access to mosquito nets, but these were usually only available to officers and hospital patients (see Post, *Soldiers' Letters*, 42).

46. Fletcher, *Rebel Private*, 32–33.

47. Ibid., 9–10.

48. Van Buren, *Rules for Preserving the Health of the Soldier*, 8.

49. Billings, *Hardtack and Coffee*, 80–82. See also Post, *Soldiers' Letters*, 42.

50. Anonymous, 11th Massachusetts Infantry, to Jim, May 20, 1862, Civil War letters of a Massachusetts 11th Soldier, UVA.

51. Carpenter, *War Diary of Kinchen Jahu Carpenter*, 8.

52. "Correspondence from 'the Army of Virginia,'" *Valley Spirit*, August 20, 1862, VSVCDH.

53. Norton, *Army Letters*, 97.

54. McCrea, *Dear Belle*, 139.

55. Blake to parents, July 9, 1862, Blake, Joseph E.—CWMiscColl, USAMHI. See also Brand to Kate, July 25, 1862, Papers of William Francis Brand, 1856–1959, UVA.

56. Haydon, *For Country, Cause & Leader*, 253.

57. Ashley to parents, June 25, 1862, Ashley Family—CWMiscColl, USAMHI. For men in the cavalry, it was even more important to camp in a location close to substantial water supplies, as they shared water with thirsty horses; see Whitehorne, "Blueprint for Nineteenth-Century Camps: Castramentation, 1778–1865," 29.

58. Bell to sister, May 27, 1862, Bell, David—Papers, USAMHI.

59. Pvt. Fred R. Laubach, 93rd Pennsylvania Infantry, diary [April 4, 1862, entry], Fred R. Laubach Co. H, 93rd Pennsylvania Diary, 1862–1865, USAMHI. See also Bellard, *Gone for a Soldier*, 58.

60. Major Jones diary [April 29, 1862, entry], Frank B. Jones Diary, March-June 1862, MOC.

61. Also see Sgt. David C. Ashley, 6th New York Calvary, letter to parents, May 31, 1862, Ashley Family—CWMiscColl (Sgt-Maj's letters, October 1861–64), USAMHI.

62. Ashley to parents, May 31, 1862, Ashley Family—CWMiscColl, USAMHI and Blackington to Hannah, June 24 and May 22, 1862, Blackington, Lyman and Jacob—BlackingtonColl, USAMHI.

63. John Bevan to parents, July 5, 1982, "Picketing along the Rappahannock," USAMHI. See also Private Wood diary [see most entries in July and August, 1862], Journal of Private Ephraim A. Wood, UVA; Corporal Blake, to parents, July 9, 1862, Blake, Joseph E.—CWMiscColl, USAMHI; and Private Smiley diary [July 22, 1862, entry], VSVCDH.

64. Private Perkins diary [August 4, 1862], Perkins, Charles C.—CWTIColl, USAMHI.

65. Holmes, *Touched with Fire*, 55.

66. Gill, *Courier for Lee and Jackson*, 16.

67. Pryor, *A Post of Honor*, 152–53.

68. Capt. Josiah C. Fuller, 32nd Massachusetts Infantry, to parents, June 29, 1862 (Captain's letters, 1862–64), Fuller, Josiah—Wiley Sword Collection, USAMHI.

69. Corporal Hands, Washington Hands Civil War Notebook, 40, UVA.

70. Sheeran, *Confederate Chaplain*, 21–22.

71. Schantz explains that death also had the ability to level the classes (Schantz, *Awaiting the Heavenly Country*, 4).

72. Private Perkins diary [May 19, 1862], Perkins, Charles C.—CWTIColl, USAMHI.

73. Stilwell, *The Stilwell Letters*, 23, 25.

74. John Bevan to parents, February 2, 1862, "Picketing along the Rappahannock," USAMHI.

75. It is important to note, however, that the men accused each other of malingering far less often than did officers at the brigade level and above.

76. Hulbert, *One Battle Too Many*, 65.

77. Stewart, *Camp, March and Battle-field*, 74.

78. Private Davis to sister Angie, August 1, 1862, A. S. Davis Civil War Letters, UVA.

79. Fitzpatrick, *Letters to Amanda*, 7.

80. Lt. John Bedingfield to Pa and Ma, July 1, 1862, Bedingfield Family Civil War Letters, UVA.

81. Trueheart, *Rebel Brothers*, 53.

82. Booth, *A Maryland Boy in Lee's Army*, 56.

83. Pvt. John O'Farrell, Crenshaw's Battery Artillery, diary [June 6, 1862, entry], John O'Farrell Diary, MOC; Fitzpatrick, *Letters to Amanda*, 13–14. For an example of a Shenandoah Valley resident repeatedly opening her home to Confederate sick, see Maria Louisa Wacker Fleet, Maria Louisa Wacker Fleet Papers, 1822–1900, LVA.

84. For example, Pvt. Ephraim Wood of the 13th Massachusetts Infantry, stationed in the Shenandoah Valley, stopped at a local house for a drink of water. A former

clockmaker, he fixed the residents' clock, lamenting that some unruly Federals had broken it in the first place (Private Wood diary [July 13, 1862, entry], Journal of Private Ephraim A. Wood, UVA).

85. Handerson, *Yankee in Gray*, 92. Likewise did Maria Louisa Wacker Fleet prepare boxes for the soldiers stationed in the Shenandoah Valley; see Fleet to "My Dear Child," March 7, 1862, Maria Louisa Wacker Fleet Papers, 1822–1900, LVA.

86. Cpl. Charles Freeman Read, 3rd Massachusetts Cavalry, memoir manuscript, 3–7, MHS.

87. Howard, *Recollections of a Maryland Confederate Soldier*, 94.

88. Fletcher, *Rebel Private*, 9–10.

89. Ashley, to parents, May 31, June 25, 1862, Ashley Family—CWMiscColl, USAMHI. In another example, Private Liscom from Massachusetts, stationed in the Valley, purchased water and flour biscuits from enslaved bakers (Albert Liscom to parents, June 13, 22, Liscom, Albert M.—CWMiscColl, USAMHI).

90. See, for instance, Pender, *The General to His Lady*, 109, in which General William D. Pender explained that his enslaved servant, Harris, attended to him in sickness.

91. Sommers, "They Fired into Us an Awful Fire," 1:145.

92. Watson to mother, January 20, Letters of David Watson 1861–62, UVA.

93. Lt. Charles Barnard Fox, 13th Massachusetts Infantry, diary [April 2, 12, 1862, entry], Charles Barnard Fox Diary, MHS.

94. Pvt. George W. Baylor requested of his sister: "I want you to send me a shirt and a pair of cotton pants in the same size off my Sunday pants. I would like to have them as soon as you can send them. I [unclear] to have a Calico shirt at home I think" (Pvt. George W. Baylor, 5th Virginia Infantry, to Mary C. Baylor, June 12, 1862, George W. and Mary C. Baylor Papers, VSVCDH). See also Brand to Kate, January 10, 1862, Papers of William Francis Brand, 1856–1959, UVA.

95. Pvt. Gerald Fitzgerald, 2nd Massachusetts Infantry, to Miss Sarah Appleton, July 16, 1862, Haven-Appleton-Cutter Papers, 1692–1972, MHS.

96. Pratt to father, June 28, 1862, Pratt, Lorenzo N.—CWMiscColl, USAMHI. See also Ashley to parents, April 31, 1862, Ashley Family—CWMiscColl, USAMHI.

97. Lystra, *Searching the Heart*, 4.

98. Sgt. John S. Willey, 1st Massachusetts Infantry, to wife, April 27, 1862, Willey, John S.—HCWRTColl-DanielsColl (Sgt/LT's letters to wife, July 14, 1861–April 24, 1864), USAMHI.

99. Pvt. Henry H. Dedrick, 52nd Virginia Infantry, to Mary E. A. Dedrick, April 7, 1862, Henry H. and Mary E. A. Dedrick Family Papers, VSVCDH.

100. Mary to Henry Dedrick, April 15, 1862, Henry H. and Mary E. A. Dedrick Family Papers, VSVCDH.

101. Sergeant West diary [February 4–8, 1862, entry], William H. West Papers, MHS. See also Watson to Mother, January 20, 1862, Letters of David Watson 1861–62, UVA.

102. Bell to sister, March 6, 1862, Bell, David—Papers, USAMHI; see also Pvt. William T. Shimp, 46th Pennsylvania, to Anna, August 13, 1862, Shimp, William T.—CWMiscColl (Enlisted man's letters, December 2, 1861–January 26, 1865; Company roster, July 16, 1865), Box 6, USAMHI.

103. McPherson, *This Mighty Scourge*, 155–56, discusses the frequency with which soldiers read newspapers.

104. "Soldier Health—Interesting Soldier Recommendation," *5th Pennsylvania*, June 10, 1861, BA.

105. "Spirit Rations for the Army," *Richmond Daily Dispatch*, June 14, 1862.

106. "The Roads—Mud and Dust," *Harper's Weekly*, June 7, 1862.

107. "Portable Soup," *Richmond Daily Dispatch*, July 15, 16, 1862, NYPL. Historian and physician Alfred J. Bollet confirms that poorly prepared food was one of the primary causes of diarrhea and dysentery (Bollet, "Scurvy and Chronic Diarrhea in Civil War Troops," 49).

108. "Soldier's Health," *Christian Recorder*, November 1, 1862. See also "Camp Diseases—How to Avoid Them," *Staunton Spectator*, February 11, 1862, VSVCDH, which conveyed such explanations and remedies as the following: "The commonest cause of diarrhea is bad water, its cure, complete rest and abstinence from every kind of food except plain boiled rice."

109. "Regimental and Brigade Hospitals," *Christian Recorder*, December 28, 1861.

110. See, for example, Steiner, *Disease in the Civil War*, 14, and Bell, *Mosquito Soldiers*, 4.

111. The combat seasoning process has been well covered by historians such as Earl J. Hess and Eric T. Dean Jr. (see Hess, *The Union Soldier in Battle*, and Dean, "Dangled over Hell").

112. Fletcher, *Rebel Private*, 16.

113. Blackford, *Letters from Lee's Army*, 96.

114. Blackington to Sister, June 10 and 24, 1862, Blackington, Lyman and Jacob— BlackingtonColl, USAMHI.

115. Morgan, *Personal Reminiscences of the War*, 100.

116. Moore, *The Story of a Cannoneer*, 44.

117. Worsham, *One of Jackson's Foot Cavalry*, 105.

118. Pryor, *A Post of Honor*, 227.

CHAPTER 5

1. This is a paradox that William Blair has also somewhat explored, writing that "straggling probably helped the army by increasing the morale of men" (*Virginia's Private*, 88).

2. A traditional line of academic analysis conflates desertion and straggling as problems of lack of devotion to cause and country. See, for instance, Mitchell, *Civil War Soldiers*, 168–71; Weitz, *More Damning Than Slaughter*, xviii–xix; and McPherson, *For Cause and Comrades*, 168. Alternately, works such as Blair, *Virginia's Private War*, 60; Carmichael, *The Last Generation*, 154–56; and Ruffner, "Civil War Desertion," 101, convincingly argue that this is a problematic oversimplification of the motivations behind desertion and straggling.

3. Peter Carmichael likewise refers to the fact that "higher military authorities refused to condone [straggling] under any circumstances" (Carmichael, *The Last Generation*, 155).

4. The improvement of logistical conditions in the late fall and winter of 1862 is something that Keith Bohannon examines for the Army of Northern Virginia in "Dirty, Ragged, and Ill-Provided For," 130–31, and George Rable investigates for the Army of the Potomac in *Fredericksburg! Fredericksburg!*, 64–65.

5. Billings, *Hardtack and Coffee*, 144.

6. Ella Lonn's detailed book presents many reasons for desertion relevant to this investigation of straggling, including lack of shoes, delayed pay, short rations, sickness, and exposure to bad weather. It is actually more common that such circumstances prompted straggling, because of their relationship to self-care (Lonn, *Desertion in the Civil War*, 8–11).

7. Weitz, *More Damning Than Slaughter*, 96. Indeed, straggling has rarely been the subject of extended analysis, is usually only referred to as a subset of desertion, and is almost never examined in the Union armies. A handful of historians have mentioned straggling and desertion as separate issues in broader works on desertion or logistical problems; see Bohannon, "Dirty, Ragged, and Ill-Provided For," 110; Carmichael, "So Far from God," 55–56; Carmichael, *The Last Generation*, 154; Glatthaar, *Lee's Army*, 140; and Blair, *Virginia's Private War*, 60–62. The most nuanced and protracted analysis of straggling as a separate problem from desertion is Harsh, *Taken at the Flood*, 44–45, 94, 117–19.

8. Linderman, *Embattled Courage*, 10. The quote is from George Cary Eggleston, a Confederate soldier.

9. Handerson, *Yankee in Gray*, 39.

10. Ibid., 39–40.

11. McKim, *A Soldier's Recollections*, 78–79.

12. Pvt. Wood diary [July 13 and 30, 1862, entries], Journal of Private Ephraim A. Wood, UVA.

13. Pvt. E. Kendall Jenkins, 1st Massachusetts Heavy Artillery, diary [August 5, 1862, entry], E. Kendall Jenkins Diaries, 1862–1879, MHS.

14. Carpenter, *War Diary of Kinchen Jahu Carpenter*, 8.

15. Private Smith diary [April 10, 1864, entry], Civil War Diary of William Randolph Smith, UVA.

16. Cpl. Horace M. Wade, 12th Virginia Cavalry, to parents, May 3, 1862, Wade, Horse M (Letters)—Leigh Collection Bk 33A, USAMHI.

17. Patterson, *Yankee Rebel*, 15–16.

18. Handerson, *Yankee in Gray*, 50.

19. Historian Peter Cozzens has noted this in the Valley as well (Cozzens, *Shenandoah 1862*, 94).

20. McClellan, *Welcome the Hour of Conflict*, 156.

21. Paxton, *Memoir and Memorials*, 58.

22. Pvt. Charles Perkins diary [March 29, April 15, and August 15, 1862, entries], Perkins, Charles C.—CWTIColl, USAMHI.

23. Keiser, *Diary of Henry Keiser of Lykens*, typescript, 30, USAMHI.

24. Sergeant West diary [February 10, March 10, April 4, 1862, entries], William H. West Papers, MHS.

25. Stilwell, *The Stilwell Letters*, 10.

26. Private Blackington to sister, June 24, 1862, Blackington, Lyman and Jacob—BlackingtonColl, USAMHI;

27. See Private Wood diary [July and August entries], Journal of Private Ephraim A. Wood, UVA.

28. Joseph Glatthaar similarly writes that "the cavalry had the highest percentage of deserters, with almost one in every five" in the Army of Northern Virginia (Glatthaar, *General Lee's Army*, 410).

29. Sergeant Ashley to parents, May 31, 1862, Ashley Family—CWMiscColl, USAMHI.

30. Peter Carmichael, for instance, writes that desertion in spring and summer of 1862 was "driven by home front needs" (Carmichael, "So Far from God," 26).

31. For example, see the Hite brothers, *I Have Painful News to Write*.

32. Haydon, *For Country, Cause & Leader*, 231.

33. *OR*, ser. 1, vol. 11, 1:605.

34. Officers were not supposed to occupy houses without express permission of brigade command (U.S. War Department, *Revised Regulations*, 76).

35. Paxton, *Memoir and Memorials*, 58.

36. Major Jones diary [March 15 and April 18, 1862, entries], Frank B. Jones Diary, March-June 1862, MOC.

37. Casler, *Four Years in the Stonewall Brigade*, 101.

38. Ibid., 50, and Billings, *Hardtack and Coffee*, 145. See also Rable, *Civil Wars*, 93.

39. Lonn, *Desertion in the Civil War*, 228; Billings, *Hardtack and Coffee*, 144–56.

40. Carmichael, "So Far from God," 43.

41. Trueheart, *Rebel Brothers*, 41–43.

42. Cozzens, *Shenandoah 1862*, 94. At this point Surgeon Hunter McGuire examined Loring's brigades and accused them of malingering, returning 1,000 men to their units without care (Robertson, *Stonewall Jackson*, 315).

43. Carmichael, "Turner Ashby's Appeal," 163–65.

44. Conscription enrolled all white men between eighteen and thirty-five except for those with legal exemptions (Glatthaar, *General Lee's Army*, 85).

45. Carmichael, "So Far from God," 38, and Blair, *Virginia Private's War*, 61, report that desertion dramatically increased following the draft, but George Rable argues the opposite. Conscription, Rable writes, "legally discharged those soldiers who were most prone to desertion: the regiment's older personnel who were physically incapable of performing military duty; the extremely young who were not psychologically prepared for war; and foreigners who never fully supported the Southern cause" (Rable, *Civil Wars*, 95).

46. Moore, *The Story of a Cannoneer*, 45–47.

47. Howard, *Recollections of a Maryland Confederate Soldier*, 78.

48. Cozzens, *Shenandoah 1862*, 421–22.

49. Worsham, *One of Jackson's Foot Cavalry*, 104–5.

50. Carmichael, "So Far from God," 46. Carmichael attributes the spike in absenteeism to this being the first time that Jackson's troops had campaigned far from home: "Emotional stress understandably mounted that summer, as [Jackson's soldiers] worried about the safety and well-being of their families."

51. Worsham, *One of Jackson's Foot Cavalry*, 104–5.

52. Sears, *To the Gates of Richmond*, 331. Straggling in Magruder's ranks resulted mainly from his own errors and those of his guide.

53. Weitz, *More Damning Than Slaughter*, 42; Blair, *Virginia's Private War*, 67.

54. Burton, *Extraordinary Circumstances*, 259–60.

55. Harsh, *Taken at the Flood*, 117.

56. *OR*, ser. 1, vol. 19, 1:143.

57. Carmichael, "So Far from God," 48. As in the case of Casler mentioned earlier, it may have even encouraged men to desert (Casler, *Four Years in the Stonewall Brigade*, 101).

58. Carmichael, "So Far from God," 53, 62. Of the Confederates arrested from July 27 to August 14, twelve percent were sentenced to death; forty percent had sentences overturned due to irregularities (Carmichael, "So Far from God," 45).

59. *OR*, ser. 4, vol. 2, 7.

60. Confederate States of America, *General Orders Numbers*, No. 94, August 11, 1862. See also Confederate States of America, "Medical Requisition and Sick Lists and General Orders 25th Regiment, Virginia Vol. 1861–64," No. 36 (May 17, 1862) and No. 78 (August 2, 1862), LVA.

61. Confederate States of America, *General Orders*, No. 137, December 28, 1862; Weitz, *More Damning Than Slaughter*, 87.

62. For instance, notes George Rable, "Desertion from the 44th Virginia Infantry Regiment was primarily a phenomenon of the early war period, a product of the recruitment of men unsuited for military life" (Rable, *Civil Wars*, 100). Mark Weitz writes that studies of smaller units of Confederate soldiers and the general observations of commanders "led to the conclusion that desertion in 1862 claimed a significant number of soldiers, making it the worst year of the war for some units. A study of ten Virginia regiments, representing four regions of the state, reveals how serious the desertion problem had become in 1862. Of the ten regiments, half had more deserters in 1862 than in any other year of the war" (Weitz, *More Damning Than Slaughter*, 94–95). Finally, Peter Carmichael explains that soon after Jackson executed three Valley soldiers in front of his men in August, discipline improved in the Second Manassas campaign. The veterans there "displayed a degree of professionalism not shown in earlier campaigns" (Carmichael, "So Far from God," 65).

63. Murray, *Witness to the Civil*, 63.

64. Cozzens, *Shenandoah 1862*, 421, 151–52, 233, 430.

65. *OR*, ser. 1, vol. 11, 1:183–85.

66. Sears, *To the Gates of Richmond*, 109.

67. McClellan, *The Civil War Papers of George B. McClellan*, 373.

68. Sears, *To the Gates of Richmond*, 337–38.

69. As an example see Gary G. Lash's investigation of the 71st Pennsylvania (Lash, "No Praise Can Be Too Good for the Officers and Men," 3:57).

70. *OR*, ser. 1, vol. 11, 3: 319.

71. Marvell, *Burnside*, 163.

72. *OR*, ser. 1, vol. 12, 2:52.

73. Lonn, *Desertion during the Civil War*, 143–4; Carmichael, "So Far from God," 45.

74. John Hunter Harrison to Surgeon General's Office, "From Your Quarterly Report of Sick and Wounded for Quarter Ending June 30, 1862," July 28, 1862, Papers of John Hunter Harrison 1842–1888, UVA.

75. *OR*, ser. 1, vol. 11, 1:206.

76. See, for example, Miller, "I Wait Only for the River," 58.

77. As historian Joseph Glatthaar concludes in his extensive study of the Army of Northern Virginia, a more consistent use of furloughs could have improved morale: "Unfortunately, both Johnston and then Lee awarded furloughs stingily. Two per one hundred men or two per company was standard practice" (Glatthaar, *General Lee's Army*, 225).

78. Both sides offered veterans furloughs to those who would reenlist. A Confederate Act of December 11, 1861, specifically provided "for the granting of bounties and furloughs to privates and non-commissioned officers in the Provisional Army" (Schwab, *The Confederate States of America*, 193).

79. *OR*, ser. 1, vol. 5, 1016, 1037.

80. Ibid., 1045.

81. Ibid., 1072, 1075.

82. *OR*, ser. 1, vol. 21, 869.

83. Cunningham, *Doctors in Gray*, 41–42.

84. *OR*, ser. 1, vol. 5, 1041.

85. *OR*, ser. 1, vol. 5, 1046–47.

86. Carmichael, *The Last Generation*, 154.

87. *OR*, ser. 1, vol. 11, 3:331.

88. *OR*, ser. 1, vol. 12, 3:262.

89. Lincoln, *The Collected Works*, 5:484.

90. Pryor, *A Post of Honor*, 131.

91. William Blair discusses the increasing propensity toward punishing deserters (Blair, *Virginia's Private War*, 55–68).

92. Private Taylor to mother, February 8, 1862, and to John H. Horsham, April 28, 1862, Papers of Charles Elisha Taylor, 1849–1874, UVA.

93. As Joseph Glatthaar's detailed statistical portrait of the Army of Northern Virginia has made clear, straggling and desertion continued to ebb and flow as the war progressed, though Glatthaar tracked mainly desertion: "The last quarter of 1862 witnessed a doubling of the desertion rate from its highest total in the fourth previous quarters. . . . Although desertion rates declined in early 1863, they increased after Chancellorsville and then reached new heights in the last half of the year." In short, he cites "an accelerating pattern of desertion, following the progress of the war" (Glatthaar, *General Lee's Army*, 412).

CONCLUSION

1. George Perkins, *Three Years a Soldier*, 47–48. Descriptions quoted and paraphrased from Pvt. George Perkins's letters, May 22–31, 1862.

2. According to Reid Mitchell's appraisal of Bell Irvin Wiley's *Johnny Reb* and *Billy Yank*, arguably the most influential works on common soldiers, the only real source of

difference Wiley was able to identify between Confederate and Union soldiers was the superior Union logistical capacity (Mitchell, "Not the General but the Soldier," 83).

3. Historian Melinda Lawson has detailed the process by which the United States used Sanitary Fairs, extensive pamphleteering, and social organizations, such as gentlemen's clubs, to incite loyalty to nation by investing concern in Union soldiers' suffering at the warfront (Lawson, *Patriot Fires*, 26–29, 98–99, 117–19). Frances Clarke also supports the idea that the United States proved particularly adept at mobilizing Northern suffering on behalf of Civil War soldiers (Clarke, *War Stories*, 2).

4. In the sense that this book portrays Union and Confederate soldiers as sharing a common cultural background, it follows in the footsteps of Reid Mitchell, *Civil War Soldiers*; Bell Irvin Wiley, *Johnny Reb* and *Billy Yank*; Gerald Linderman, *Embattled Courage*; and Randall Jimseron, *The Private Civil War*.

5. "Sanitary Statistics of the Army: Interesting Facts of the War Developed by the U.S. Sanitary Commission," April 16, 1862, *Chicago Tribune*.

6. Batholow, "The Various Influences," 8, 11.

7. Consider again this from Wayland F. Dunaway's 1913 memoir: "General Johnston posted his army between Richmond and the Chickahominy river . . . in the pestilential low-grounds of that sluggish stream. Swarms of mosquitoes attacked us at night and with their hypodermic proboscides injected poisonous malaria in our veins, to avoid which the sleeping soldier covered his head with a blanket. The complexion of the men became sallow, and every day numbers of the men were put on the sick-list by the surgeons" (Dunaway, *Reminiscences of a Rebel*, 23).

Bibliography

PRIMARY SOURCES

Archival Materials

Boston Athenaeum Special Collections, Boston, Massachusetts
 George W. Allen Diary
 Confederate Imprints Collection
 Confederate Subsistence Ledgers, 1862–1863
 Hugh Cummings Diary
 Robert B. Smith Letters
Library of Virginia, Archives and Manuscripts, Richmond, Virginia
 25th Virginia Infantry Regiment, Medical Records, 1861–1865
 James Richmond Boulware Diary
 G. Q. French Diary
 Ivory Family Letters
 Maria Louisa Wacker Fleet Papers
 Civil War Papers of Edward Rush Young
Massachusetts Historical Society, Boston, Massachusetts
 Bailey family Letters
 Charles Barnard Fox Diary
 Henry Bellows Papers
 William Sturgis Bigelow Papers
 Charles Henry Dalton Correspondence
 War Papers of Frank B. Fay
 James B. Fry Report
 Samuel A. Green Papers
 Haven-Appleton-Cutter Papers
 William Clark Hawes Diary
 John Theodore Heard Papers
 E. Kendall Jenkins Diaries
 Frederick Newman Knapp Papers
 Asa Farnsworth Lawrence Paper
 James W. Paige Papers
 Charles Freeman Read Diary
 Diaries of Henry Bromfield Rogers
 Lewis C. Shepard Diary
 Asa D. Smith Diary
 David Thayer Papers

Tufts-Robertson Papers
United States Sanitary Commission Camp Inspection Returns
United States Sanitary Commission Reports of Committees
William H. West Papers
Alfred Metcalf White Letters
Military History Institute, U.S. Army War College, Carlisle, Pennsylvania
Edward A. Acton Letters
George L. Andrews Papers
Ashley Family Papers
Aaron E. Bachman Memoir
David Bell Papers
Allen L. and John H. Bevan Letters
George Bills Letters
W. H. Bird Memoir
Eugene Blackford Papers
Lyman & Jacob Blackington Papers
Joseph E. Blake Letters
Alvin N. Brackett Letters
John Brislin Letters
George Clark Memoir
Samuel A. Craig Memoir
Civil War Letters of James Crane
Arnold P. Dains Letters
John C. Ellis Letters
Josiah C. Fuller Letter
John M. Fullerton Letters
Jacob W. Haas Papers
Diary of Henry Keiser
Jacob Kiester Correspondence
Thomas Landers Letters
Benjamin Landon Diary
Thomas Langstroth Letters
Philip A. Lantzy Letters
Fred R. Laubach Diary
Henry Lieb Diary
Albert Liscom Letters
Henry Lyle Correspondence
Lewis J. Martin Letters
James H. McIlwain Letters
George W. Mindil Papers
William H. Myers Letters
George Washington Newmyer Letter
Charles C. Perkins Diaries
Lorenzo N. Pratt Letters
Frasier Rosenkrans Letters

William T. Shimp Letters
Valentine W. Southall Letters
Thomas Taylor Diary
Horace M. Wade Letters
John S. Willey Letters
Museum of the Confederacy, Richmond, Virginia
Robert G. Halloway Diary
Hunter Holmes McGuire Collection
Frank B. Jones Diary
Merriwether Lewis Letters
Benjamin T. Marvin Diary
Medical Personnel Collection
Marx Mitteldorfer Letters
John O' Farrell Diary
Sally Louisa Tompkins and Robertson Hospital Collection
New York Public Library—Humanities and Social Sciences, Manuscripts and
        Archives Division, New York City, New York
    U.S. Sanitary Commission Records, 1861–1878, Miscellaneous Collection
        American Association for the Relief of the Misery of Battle Fields, 1866–1870
        Condensed Historical Matter
        English Branch Archives, 1864–1865
        Medical Committee Archives, 1861–1866
        Statistical Bureau Archives. Camp Inspection Returns, 1861–1864
        Washington Hospital Directory Archives
University of Virginia, Special Collections, Charlottesville, Virginia
    Anonymous Civil War Letters of an 11th Massachusetts Soldier
    Bedingfield Family Civil War letters
    Henry T. Blanchard Letter
    Papers of William Francis Brand
    Allen Seymour Davis Papers
    John Carpenter Eakle Letter
    Civil War Diary of Irwin C. Fox
    Civil War Diary of Wesley A. Hammond
    Papers of John Hunter Harrison
    Papers of Jedediah Hotchkiss
    Notebook of Robert Thurston Hubard
    Civil War Letters to Mary Hutchinson
    Papers of the Jones Family of Louisa County
    Letter Book of John Leavitt
    Reuben Manning Newman Diary
    W. H. Redman Papers
    Civil War Diary of William Randolph Smith
    Papers of Charles Elisha Taylor
    David Watson Letters
    William Riddick Whitehead Memoir

Papers of James Peter Williams
Journal of Private Ephraim A. Wood
Valley of the Shadow: Two Communities in the American Civil War, University of
        Virginia (World Wide Web)
Diary of Harvey Bear
Diary of James E. Beard
Letters of the Brooks Family
James Carman Papers
Henry H. Dedrick Letters
Diary of Nancy Emerson
Letters of Annie Harris
Jedediah Hotchkiss Papers
Kersh Family Papers
Letters of the McCutchan Family
Letters of the Smiley Family

Newspapers

Alexandria Gazette	*National ERA*
Cavalier	*New York Herald*
Chicago Tribune	*New York Post*
Christian Banner	*New York Times*
Christian Recorder	*Richmond Daily Dispatch*
Colored American	*Richmond Enquirer*
Day Book	*Richmond Whig*
Fifth Pennsylvania	*Semi-Weekly Dispatch*
Frank Leslie's Illustrated Newspaper	*Staunton Spectator*
Harper's Weekly	*Valley Spirit*
Maryland News Sheet	

Government Documents

Confederate States of America. *Army Regulations, Adopted for Use by the Confederate Army*. Richmond: West & Johnson, 1861.

———. *Almanac and Repository of Useful Knowledge, 1862*. Vicksburg, Miss: H. C. Clarke, 1861.

———. *Almanac and Repository of Useful Knowledge, 1863*. Augusta, Ga.: H. C. Clarke, 1863.

———. *Reports of the Operations of the Army of Northern Virginia from June 1862*. Richmond: R. M. Smith, 1864.

Confederate States of America, Army Medical Department. *Regulations for the Medical Department of the Confederate Army*. Richmond: Ritchie and Dunnavant, 1861.

Confederate States of America, Army of Northern Virginia. *General Orders*. Richmond: Confederate States of America, 1862.

Confederate States of America, Congress House of Representatives. *A Bill to Regulate Furloughs and Discharges to Soldiers in Hospitals*. Richmond: Confederate States of America, 1863.

———. *Report of Hospital Committee*. Richmond: Confederate States of America, 1862.

Gilham, William. *Manual of Instruction for the Volunteers and Militia of the United States*. Philadelphia: Charles Desilver, 1861.

U.S. War Department. *The Medical and Surgical History of the War of the Rebellion: Prepared, in Accordance with the Acts of Congress, Under the Direction of Surgeon General Joseph K. Barnes, United States Army*. 6 vols., index and illustrations. Washington, D.C.: Government Printing Office, 1870–88.

———. *The War of the Rebellion: A Compilation of the Official Records of the Union and Confederate Armies*. 127 vols., index and atlas. Washington, D.C.: Government Printing Office, 1880–1901.

———. *Revised Regulations for the Army of the United States, 1861*. Philadelphia: J. G. L. Brown, Printer, 1861.

Published Medical Sources

American Citizen. *The Philanthropic Results of the War in America: Collected from Official and Other Authentic Sources*. New York: Press of Wynkoop, Hallenbeck & Thomas, 1863.

Batholow, Robert. "The Various Influences Affecting the Physical Endurance, the Power of Resisting Disease, etc., of the Men Composing the Volunteer Armies of the United States." In *Contributions Relating to the Causation and Prevention of Disease, and to Camp Diseases*, ed. Austin Flint, 3–41. New York: Hurd and Houghton, 1867.

Buchan, William. *Domestic Medicine: Or a Treatise for the Prevention and Cure of Diseases, by Regimen and Simple Medicines*. 1801. Reprint, Halifax: Milner and Sowerby, 1859.

Campbell, David, ed. *The Graham Journal of Health and Longevity Devoted to the Practical Illustration of the Science of Human Life, as Taught by Sylvester Graham and Others*. 3 vols. Boston: George P. Oakes, April 1837–December 1839.

Drake, Daniel. "Selected Papers: Medical Topography. From the Natural and Statistical View, or Picture of Cincinnati and the Miami Country." *Eclectic Repertory and Analytical Review, Medical and Philosophical* 6 (April 1816): 137.

Flint, Austin. *Contributions Relating to the Causation and Prevention of Disease, and to Camp Diseases*. New York: Hurd and Houghton, 1867.

Gould, Benjamin Apthorp. *United States Sanitary Commission Memoirs: Statistical or Investigations in the Military and Anthropological Statistics of American Soldiers*. New York: Hurd and Houghton, 1869.

Greenleaf, Charles R. *A Manual for the Medical Officers of the United States Army*. 1864. Reprint, San Francisco: Norman, 1992.

Gunn, John C. *Gunn's Domestic Medicine*. 1830. Reprint, New York: C. M. Saxton, Barber, 1860.

Hippocrates. *On Water, Airs, and Places: The Received Greek Text of Littré, with Latin, French, and English Translations by Eminent Scholars*. London: Wyman & Sons, 1881.

Lucas, Charles S. "Observations on the Medical Topography and Endemic Fever of Montgomery County, Alabama." *American Journal of the Medical Sciences* 1 (November 1827): 78.

MacDonough, Augustus R. et al. *The Spirit of the Fair: None but the Brave Deserve the Fair*. New York: John F. Trow, 1864.

Metcalfe, John T. *Report of a Committee of the Associate Members of the United States Sanitary Commission, On the Subject of the Nature and Treatment of Miasmatic Fevers*. New York: Baillière Brothers, 1862.

Ordronaux, John. *Manual of Instructions for Military Surgeons: On the Examination of Recruits and Discharge of Soldiers*. New York: D. Van Nostrand, 1863.

"The Pathology and Treatment of Periodical Fevers." *Boston Medical and Surgical Journal* 37 (December 1847): 378.

Post, Alfred C., and William H. Van Buren. *Report on Military Hygiene and Therapeutics*. 1861. Reprint, Washington, D.C.: Sanitary Commission, 1863.

Ray, Issac. *Mental Hygiene*. 1863. Reprint, New York: Hafner Publishing, 1968.

Somervail, Alexander. "On the Medical Topography and Diseases of a Section of Virginia." *Philadelphia Journal of the Medical and Physical Sciences* 6 (April 1823): 276.

Stillé, Charles Janeway. *History of the United States Sanitary Commission: Being the General Report of Its Work Done during the War of the Rebellion*. Philadelphia: J. B. Lippincott, 1866.

Strong, G. T. *Origin, Struggles and Principles of the U.S. Sanitary Commission*. Boston: s.n., 1864.

Suckley, George, J. G. Cooper, et al. *The Natural History of Washington Territory: with much relating to Minnesota, Nebraska, Kansas, Oregon, and California, between the thirty-sixth and forty-ninth parallels of latitude, being those parts of the final reports on the survey of the Northern Pacific railroad route, containing the climate and physical geography, with full catalogues and descriptions of the plants and animals collected from 1853 to 1857*. New York: Baillière Brothers, 1859.

Swinburne, John. *Reports on the Peninsular Campaign, Surgical Experience*. Albany, N.Y.: Steam Press of C. Van Benthuysen, 1863.

Thomson, James W. "An Inquiry into the Medical Topography and Epidemic Fevers of the Valley of Virginia." *Philadelphia Journal of the Medical and Physical Sciences* 1 (January 1825): 96.

"Traveling editorials." *Western Journal of Medicine and Surgery* 7 (June 1843): 469.

United States Sanitary Commission. *The American Association for the Relief of the Misery of Battle fields: A Central National Committee . . . Constituted by an International Conference at Geneva, Switzerland in Oct. 1863*. Washington, D.C.: Gibson Brothers, 1866.

———. *Branch of the U.S. Sanitary Commission, First Annual Report of the Women's Central Association of Relief May 1, 1862*. New York: William C. Bryant, 1862.

———. *Documents of the U.S. Sanitary Commission*. 3 vols. New York: s.n., 1856–1866.

———. *Hints for the Control and Prevention of Infectious Diseases: In Camps, Transports, and Hospitals.* New York: William C. Bryant, 1863.

———. "Object of the Examination: The Object of These Examinations Is to Ascertain the Effect of Climate, Locality, and Mode of Life upon Men 1862." S.l.: s.n., 1862.

———. *Report of a Committee . . . on Dysentery.* 2nd ed. Washington, D.C.: McGill and Witherow, 1863.

———. *Report of a Committee. . . . on the Subject of Scurvy with Special Reference to the Army and Navy.* 2nd ed. Washington, D.C.: Witherow, 1863.

———. *Report of the Secretary with Regard to the Probable Origin of the Recent Demoralization of the Volunteer Army at Washington.* Washington, D.C.: McGill and Witherow, 1861.

———. *The Sanitary Commission Bulletin.* 40 vols. New York: Sanitary Commission, 1863–1865.

———. *The Soldier's Friend.* Philadelphia: Perkinpine & Higgins, 1865.

Van Buren, William H. *Report of a Committee Appointed by Resolution of the Sanitary Commission, to Prepare a Paper on the Use of Quinine as a Prophylactic against Malarious Disease.* New York: William C. Bryant, 1861.

———. *Rules for Preserving the Health of the Soldier.* Washington, D.C.: U.S. Sanitary Commission, 1861.

Woodward, Joseph Janvier. *Outlines of the Chief Camp Diseases of the United States Armies: As Observed during the Present War.* Philadelphia: Lippincott, 1863.

Published Narratives

Alexander, Edward Porter. *Fighting for the Confederacy: The Personal Recollections of General Edward Porter Alexander.* Ed. Gary W. Gallagher. Chapel Hill: University of North Carolina Press, 1989.

Anderson, Carter S. *Train Running for the Confederacy, 1861–1865, An Eyewitness Memoir.* Ed. Walbrook D. Swank. Charlottesville, Va.: Papercraft, 1990.

Apperson, John Samuel. *Repairing the March of Mars: The Civil War Diaries of John Samuel Apperson, Hospital Steward in the Stonewall Brigade, 1861–1865.* Ed. John Herbert Roper. Macon, Ga.: Mercer Press, 2001.

Averell, William Woods. *Ten Years in the Saddle: The Memoir of William Woods Averell.* Ed. Edward K. Eckert and Nicholas J. Amato. San Rafael, Calif.: Presidio Press, 1978.

Bacot, Ada W. *A Confederate Nurse: The Diary of Ada W. Bacot, 1860–1863.* Columbia: University of South Carolina Press, 1994.

Beall, John Yates. *Memoir of John Yates Beall: His Life, Trial, Correspondence, Diary, and Private Manuscript Found among His Papers, Including His Own Account of the Raid on Lake Erie.* Ed. Daniel Bedinger Lucas. Montreal: John Lovell, 1865.

Beers, Fannie A. *Memories: A Record of Personal Experiences and Adventure during Four Years of War.* Philadelphia: Lippincott, 1888.

Bellard, Alfred. *Gone for a Soldier: The Civil War Memoirs of Private Alfred Bellard.* Ed. David Herbert Donald. Boston: Little, Brown, 1975.

Billings, John D. *Hardtack and Coffee: The Unwritten Story of Army Life*. 1887. Reprint, Lincoln: University of Nebraska Press, 1993.

Blackford, Charles Minor. *Letters from Lee's Army or Memoirs of Life in and out of the Army in Virginia during the War between the States*. Ed. Susan Leigh Blackford and Charles Minor Blackford III. New York: Charles Scribner's Sons, 1947.

Booth, G. W. *A Maryland Boy in Lee's Army: Personal Reminiscences of a Maryland Soldier in the War between the States, 1861–1865*. Ed. Eric J. Mink. Lincoln: University of Nebraska Press, 2000.

Brinton, John H. *Personal Memoirs of John H. Brinton: Civil War Surgeon, 1861–1865*. New York: Neale, 1914.

Brown, Campbell. *Campbell Brown's Civil War: With Ewell and the Army of Northern Virginia*. Ed. Terry L. Jones. Baton Rouge: Louisiana State University Press, 2001.

Carpenter, Kinchen Jahu. *War Diary of Kinchen Jahu Carpenter: Company I, Fiftieth North Carolina Regiment War between the States 1861–5*. Ed. Julie Carpenter Williams. Rutherford, N.C.: s.n., 1955.

Carter, Robert Goldthwaite. *Four Brothers in Blue: Or Sunshine and Shadows of the War of the Rebellion, a Story of the Great Civil War from Bull Run to Appomattox*. Ed. John M. Carroll. Austin: University of Texas Press, 1978.

Casler, John O. *Four Years in the Stonewall Brigade*, 2nd ed. 1906. Reprint, Columbia: University of South Carolina Press, 2005.

Castleman, Alfred Lewis. *Diary of Alfred Lewis Castleman, May, 1862, in the Army of the Potomac, Behind the Scenes*. Milwaukee: Strickland, 1863.

Comey, Henry Newton. *A Legacy of Valor: The Memoirs and Letters of Captain Henry Newton Comey, 2nd Massachusetts Infantry*. Ed. Lyman Richard Comey. Knoxville: University of Tennessee Press, 2004.

Cooke, John Esten. *Wearing of the Gray; Being Personal Portraits, Scenes and Adventures of the War*. New York: E. B. Treat, 1867.

Craighill, E. A. *Confederate Surgeon: The Personal Recollections of E. A. Craighill*. Ed. Peter W. Houck. Lynchburg, Va.: H. E. Howard, 1989.

Crowther, James E. *The Crowther Letters: Family, Companions, and Rebels*. Ed. Bob Hileman Jr. 2001. Reprint, Tarentum, Pa.: Hileman House, 2004.

Cumming, Kate. *The Journal of a Confederate Nurse*. Ed. Richard Barksdale Harwell. Baton Rouge: Louisiana State University Press, 1998.

Dewey, Orville. *Autobiography and Letters of Orville Dewey, D.D.* Ed. Mary E. Dewey. Boston: Roberts Brothers, 1883.

Dunaway, Wayland. *Rev. Wayland Fuller Dunaway, Reminiscences of a Rebel*. New York: Neale Publishing Co., 1913.

Dwight, Wilder. *Life and Letters of Wilder Dwight, Lieut.–Colonel Second Massachusetts Infantry Volunteers*. Boston: Ticknor, 1891.

Dyer, J. Franklin. *The Journal of a Civil War Surgeon*. Ed. Michael B. Chesson. Lincoln: University of Nebraska Press, 2003.

Edmonds, Sarah Emma. *Memoirs of a Soldier, Nurse and Spy: A Women's Adventures in the Union Army*. DeKalb: Northern Illinois University Press, 1999.

Ellis, Thomas T. *Leaves from the Diary of an Army Surgeon: Or Incidents of Field, Camp, and Hospital Life*. New York: John Bradburn, 1863.

Everson, Erastus W. *Stories of Our Soldiers: War Reminiscences, by "Carleton" and by Soldiers of New England*. Boston: Journal Newspaper Company, 1893.

Figg, Royall W. *"Where Men Only Dare to Go!" The Story of a Boy Company.* Richmond: Whittet & Shipperson, 1885.

Fitzpatrick, Marion Hill. *Letters to Amanda: The Civil War Letters of Marion Hill Fitzpatrick, Army of Northern Virginia*. Ed. Jeffrey C. Low and Sam Hodges. Macon, Ga.: Mercer University Press, 1998.

Fletcher, William Andrew. *Rebel Private: Front and Rear*. Ed. Bell Irvin Wiley. Austin: University of Texas Press, 1954.

Gache, Louis-Hippolyte. *A Frenchman, a Chaplain, a Rebel: The War Letters of Pere Louis-Hippolyte Gache, S.J.* Ed. Cornelius M. Buckley. Chicago: Loyola University Press, 1981.

Giles, Val C. *Rags and Hope: The Recollections of Val C. Giles, Four Years with Hood's Brigade, Fourth Texas Infantry 1861-1865*. Ed. Mary Lasswell. New York: Coward-McCann, 1961.

Gill, John. *Courier for Lee and Jackson, 1861-1865 Memoirs*. Ed. Walbrook D. Swank. Shippensburg, Pa.: Burd Street Press, 1993.

Grimes, Bryan. *Extracts of Letters of Maj. Gen. Bryan Grimes to His Wife*. Raleigh, N.C.: A. Williams, 1884.

Handerson, Henry E. *Yankee in Gray: The Civil War Memoirs of Henry E. Handerson with a Selection of His Wartime Letters*. Ed. Clyde Lottride Cummer. Cleveland: Press of Western Reserve University, 1962.

Haydon, Charles B. *For Country, Cause & Leader: The Civil War Journal of Charles B. Haydon*. Ed. Stephen W. Sears. New York: Ticknor & Fields, 1993.

Hentz, Charles A. *A Southern Practice: The Diary and Autobiography of Charles A. Hentz, M.D.* Ed. Steven M. Stowe. Charlottesville: University Press of Virginia, 2000.

Hite Brothers. *The Painful News I Have to Write: Letters and Diaries of Four Hite Brothers of Page County in the Service of the Confederacy*. Ed. Harlan R. Jessup. Baltimore: Butternut & Blue, 1998.

Holmes, Oliver Wendell. *Touched with Fire: Civil War Letters and Diary of Oliver Wendell Holmes, Jr. 1861-1864*. Ed. Mark De Wolfe Howe. Cambridge, Mass.: Harvard University Press, 1947.

Holt, Daniel M. *A Surgeon's Civil War: The Letters and Diary of Daniel M. Holt, M.D.* Ed. James M. Greiner, Janet L. Coryell, and James R. Smither. Kent, Oh.: Kent State University Press, 1994.

Howard, McHenry. *Recollections of a Maryland Confederate Soldier and Staff Officer under Johnston, Jackson and Lee*. Baltimore: Williams & Wilkins, 1914.

Howe, Samuel Gridley. *Letters and Journals of Samuel Gridley Howe: The Servant of Humanity*. Ed. Laura E. Richards. Boston: Dana Estes, 1909.

Howland, Eliza Newton Woolsey. *Letters of a Family during the War for the Union 1861-1865*, ed. Georgeanna Woolsey Bacon and Eliza Woolsey Howland. New Haven, Conn.: Tuttle, Morehouse & Taylor, 1899.

Huffman, James. *Ups and Downs of a Confederate Soldier, 10th Virginia Infantry, C.S.A.* New York: William E. Rudge's Sons, 1940.

Hulbert, Simon B. *One Battle Too Many: The Writings of Simon Bolivar Hulbert Private, Company E 100th Regiment, New York State Volunteers 1861–1864*. Ed. Richard P. Galloway. Gaithersburg, Md.: Olde Soldier Books, 1987.

Johnston, Joseph Eggleston. *Narrative of Military Operations Directed during the Late War between the States*. 1874. Reprint, Bloomington: Indiana University Press, 1959.

Kearney, Philip. *Letters from the Peninsula: The Civil War Letters of General Philip Kearny*. Ed. William B. Styple. Kearny, N.J.: Belle Grove, 1988.

Ladley, Oscar. *Hearth and Knapsack: The Ladley Letters, 1857–1880*. Ed. Carl M. Becker and Ritchie Thomas. Athens: Ohio University Press, 1988.

Le Duc, William G. *Recollections of a Civil War Quartermaster: The Autobiography of William G. Le Duc*. St. Paul, Minn.: North Central, 1963.

Lee, Robert E. *Circular: Headquarters Armies of the Confederate States*. Richmond: Confederate States of America, 1865.

———. *Lee's Dispatches: Unpublished Letters of General Robert E. Lee, C.S.A., to Jefferson Davis and the War Department of the Confederate States of America, 1862–5*. Ed. Douglas Southall Freeman. New York: Knickerbocker, 1915.

———. *The Wartime Papers of Robert E. Lee*. Ed. Clifford Dowdey. New York: Da Capo Press, 1960.

Letterman, Jonathan. *Memoir of Jonathan Letterman*. Ed. Bennett A. Clements. New York: G. P. Putnam's Sons, 1883.

Lincoln, Abraham. *The Collected Works of Abraham Lincoln*. 9 vols. Ed. Roy P. Basler. New Brunswick, N.J.: Rutgers University Press, 1953–55.

Livermore, Mary A. *My Story of the War: A Woman's Narrative of Four Years Personal Experience as Nurse in the Union Army*. Hartford, Conn.: A. D. Worthington, 1890.

Longstreet, James. *From Manassas to Appomattox: Memoirs of the Civil War in America*. 1896. Reprint, Philadelphia: J.B. Lippincott Company, 1903.

Lusk, William Thompson. *War Letters of William Thompson Lusk, Captain, Assistant Adjutant-General, United States Volunteers, 1861–1865*. New York: Privately Printed, 1911.

McCarthy, Carlton. *Detailed Minutiae of Soldier Life in the Army of Northern Virginia, 1861–1865*. Lincoln: University of Nebraska Press, 1993.

McClellan, Bailey George. *I Saw the Elephant: Company D, 10th Alabama*. Ed. Norman E. Rourke. Shippensburg, Pa.: White Man Publishing Company, 1995.

McClellan, George B. *The Civil War Papers of George B. McClellan: Selected Correspondences, 1860–1865*. Ed. Stephen Sears. New York: Ticknor & Fields, 1989.

———. *McClellan's Own Story: The War for the Union, the Soldiers Who Fought It, the Civilians Who Directed It, and His Relations to It and to Them*. New York: Charles L. Webster & Company, 1887.

McClellan, William Cowan. *Welcome the Hour of Conflict: William Cowan McClellan and the 9th Alabama*. Ed. John C. Carter. Tuscaloosa: University of Alabama Press, 2007.

McCrea, Tully. *Dear Belle: Letters from a Cadet & Officer to His Sweetheart, 1858–1865*. Ed. Catherine S. Crary. Middletown, Conn.: Wesleyan University Press, 1965.

McKim, Randolph. *A Soldier's Recollections: Leaves from the Diary of a Young Confederate*. New York: Longmans, Green, 1910.

Miller, James T. *Bound to Be a Soldier: The Letters of Private James T. Miller, 111th Pennsylvania Infantry, 1861–1864*. Ed. Jedediah Mannis and Galen R. Wilson. Knoxville: University of Tennessee Press, 2001.

Monteiro, Aristides. *War Reminiscences by the Surgeon of Mosby's Command*. Richmond: C. N. Williams, 1890.

Moore, Edward A. *The Story of a Cannoneer under Stonewall Jackson: In Which Is Told the Part Taken by the Rockbridge Artillery in the Army of Northern Virginia*. Lynchburg, Va.: J. P. Bell, 1910.

Morgan, William H. *Personal Reminiscences of the War 1861–5: In Camp—en Bivouac—on the March—on Picket—on the Skirmish Line—on the Battlefield—and in Prison*. Lynchburg, Va.: J. P. Bell, 1911.

Morse, Charles Fessenden. *Letters Written during the Civil War, 1861–1865*. Privately published, 1898.

Newhall, Walter S. *Walter S. Newhall: A Memoir*. Ed. Sarah Butler Wister. Philadelphia: Caxton Press of C. Sherman, Son, 1864.

Norton, Oliver Wilcox. *Army Letters 1861–1865, Private Eighty-third Regiment Pennsylvania Vol., First Lieut. Eight U.S.C.T.* Chicago: O. L. Deming, 1903.

Olmsted, Frederick Law. *The Papers of Frederick Law Olmsted*. 7 vols. Ed. Charles E. Beveridge. Baltimore: Johns Hopkins University Press, 1977.

Olmsted, Frederick Law, and Laura L. Behling. *Hospital Transports: A Memoir of the Embarkation of the Sick and Wounded from the Peninsula of Virginia in the Summer of 1862*. Boston: Ticknor and Fields, 1863.

Patterson, Edmund DeWitt. *Yankee Rebel: The Civil War Journal of Edmund DeWitt Patterson*. Ed. John G. Barrett. Knoxville: University of Tennessee Press, 2004.

Paxton, Elisha Franklin. *Memoir and Memorials: Elisha Franklin Paxton, Brigadier-General, C. S. A., Composed of His Letters from Camp and Field While an Officer in the Confederate Army*. Ed. John Gallatin Paxton. New York: Neale, 1905.

Pember, Phoebe Yates. *A Southern Woman's Story*. Ed. George C. Rable. Columbia: University of South Carolina Press, 2002.

Pender, William Dorsey. *The General to His Lady: The Civil War Letters of William Dorsey Pender to Fanny Pender*. Chapel Hill: University of North Carolina Press, 1965.

Perkins, Charles C. "'They Fired into Us an Awful Fire': The Civil War Diary of Pvt. Charles C. Perkins, 1st Massachusetts Infantry Regiment, June 4–July 4, 1862." Ed. Richard J. Sommers. In *The Peninsula Campaign of 1862: Yorktown to the Seven Days*, 3 vols., ed. William J. Miller, 1:143–76. Campbell, Calif.: Savas Woodbury, 1993.

Perkins, George. *Three Years a Soldier: The Diary and Newspaper Correspondence of Private George Perkins, Sixth New York Independent Battery, 1861–1864*. Ed. Richard N. Griffin. Knoxville: University of Tennessee Press, 2006.

Perry, John Gardner. *Letters from a Surgeon of the Civil War*. Ed. Martha Derby. Boston: Little, Brown, 1906.

Post, Lydia Minturn. Ed. *Soldiers' Letters: From Camp, Battlefield and Prison*. New York: Bunce & Huntington, 1865.

Potter, A. *Notes of Hospital Life, from November 1861 to August 1863*. Philadelphia: Lippincott, 1863.

Pryor, S. G. *A Post of Honor: The Pryor Letters, 1861–63, Letters from Captain S. G. Pryor Twelfth Georgia Regiment and His Wife Penelope Tyson Pryor*. Ed. Charles R. Adams Jr. Fort Valley, Ga.: Garret Publications, 1989.

Putnam, Sally A. *Richmond during the War*. New York: G. W. Carleton, 1867.

Reed, William Howell. *Hospital Life in the Army of the Potomac*. Boston: William V. Spencer, 1866.

Sheeran, James B. *Confederate Chaplain: A War Journal of Rev. James B. Sheeran*. Ed. Joseph T. Durkin. Milwaukee: Bruce, 1960.

Shelton, Amanda. *Turn Backward, O Time: The Civil War Diary of Amanda Shelton*. Ed. Kathleen S. Hanson. Iowa City: Edinborough Press, 2006.

Small, Abner. *The Road to Richmond: The Civil War Memoirs of Major Abner R. Small of the 16th Maine Volunteers; Together with the Diary Which He Kept When He Was a Prisoner of War*. Ed. Harold Adams Small. Berkeley: University of California Press, 1939.

Smith, William Mervale. *Swamp Doctor: The Diary of a Union Surgeon in the Virginia and North Carolina Marshes*. Ed. Thomas P Lowry. Mechanicsburg, Pa.: Stackpole Books, 2001.

Stewart, A. M. *Camp, March and Battle-field; on Three Years and a Half with the Army of the Potomac*. Philadelphia: Jasper B. Rodgers, 1865.

Stilwell, William R. *The Stilwell Letters: A Georgian in Longstreet's Corps, Army of Northern Virginia*. Ed. Ronald H. Moseley. Macon, Ga.: Mercer University Press, 2002.

Strother, David Hunter. *A Virginia Yankee in the Civil War: The Diaries of David Hunter Strother*. Ed. Cecil D. Eby Jr. Chapel Hill: University of North Carolina Press, 1961.

Sumner, Charles. *The Selected Letters of Charles Sumner*. 2 vols. Ed. Beverly Wilson Palmer. Boston: Northeastern University Press, 1990.

Thompson, Gilbert. *The Engineer Battalion in the Civil War. A Contribution to the History of the United States Engineers*. Washington, D.C.: Press of the Engineer School, 1910.

Thompson, James Thomas. "A Georgia Boy with 'Stonewall' Jackson: The Letters of James Thomas Thompson." *Virginia Magazine of History and Biography* 70 (July 1962): 314–31.

Trueheart, Charles William, and Henry Martyn. *Rebel Brothers: The Civil War Letters of the Truehearts*. Ed. Edward B. Williams. College Station: Texas A&M University Press, 1995.

Twichell, Joseph Hopkins. *The Civil War Letters of Joseph Hopkins Twichell: A Chaplain's Story*. Ed. Peter Messent and Steve Courtney. Athens: University of Georgia Press, 2006.

Warfield, Edgar. *Manassas to Appomattox: The Civil War Memoirs of Pvt. Edgar Warfield, 17th Infantry*. McLean, Va.: EPM Publications, 1996.

Watson, William. *Letters of a Civil War Surgeon*. Ed. Paul Fatout. West Lafayette, Ind.: Purdue University Press, 1996.

Welch, Spencer Glasgow. *A Confederate Surgeon's Letters to His Wife*. Marietta, Ga.: Continental, 1954.

Winkler, E. T. *Duties of the Citizen Soldier: A Sermon Delivered in the 1st Baptist Church of Charleston, S.C., on Sabbath Morning Jan. 6, 1861*. Charleston: A. J. Burke, 1861.

Wood, Thomas Fanning. *Doctor to the Front: The Recollections of Confederate Surgeon Thomas Fanning Wood, 1861–1865*. Ed. Donald B. Koonce. Knoxville: University of Tennessee Press, 2000.

Worsham, John H. *One of Jackson's Foot Cavalry: His Experience and What He Saw during the War 1861–1865: Including a History of "F Company." Richmond, Va., 21st Regiment Virginia Infantry, Second Brigade, Jackson's Division, Second Corps, A.N. Va.* 1912. Reprint, Alexandria, Va.: Time-Life Books, 1982.

SECONDARY WORKS

Books

Adams, George Worthington. *Doctors in Blue: The Medical History of the Union Army in the Civil War*. 1952. Reprint, Baton Rouge: Louisiana State University Press, 1996.

Allan, William. *History of the Campaign of Gen. T. J. (Stonewall) Jackson in the Shenandoah Valley of Virginia, from November 4, 1861, to June 17, 1862*. Dayton, Ohio: Morningside Bookshop, 1974.

Anderson, Fred. *A People's Army: Massachusetts Soldiers and Society in the Seven Years' War*. Chapel Hill: University of North Carolina Press, 1996.

Ashburn, P. M. *A History of the Medical Department of the United States Army*. Boston: Houghton Mifflin, 1929.

Attie, Jeanie. *Patriotic Toil: Northern Women and the American Civil War*. Ithaca, N.Y.: Cornell University Press, 1998.

Barry, John M. *The Great Influenza: The Epic Story of the Deadliest Plague in History*. New York: Viking, 2004.

Barton, Michael, and Larry M. Logue, eds. *The Civil War Soldier: A Historical Reader*. New York: New York University Press, 2002.

Bell, Andrew M. *Mosquito Soldiers: Malaria, Yellow Fever, and the Course of the American Civil War*. Baton Rouge: Louisiana State University Press, 2010.

Berry, Stephen. *All That Makes a Man: Love and Ambition in the Civil War South*. Oxford: Oxford University Press, 2003.

Black, Brian. *Nature and the Environment in 19th-Century American Life*. Westport, Conn.: Greenwood Press, 2006.

Blair, William. *Virginia's Private War: Feeding Body and Soul in the Confederacy, 1861–1865*. New York: Oxford University Press, 1998.

Bollet, Alfred J. *Civil War Medicine: Challenges and Triumphs*. Tucson, Ariz.: Galen Press, 2002.

Brady, Lisa M. *War upon the Land: Military Strategy and the Transformation of Southern Landscapes during the American Civil War*. Athens: University of Georgia Press, 2012.

Brown, Kathleen M. *Foul Bodies: Cleanliness in Early America*. New Haven, Conn.: Yale University Press, 2009.

Brown, Thomas J. *Dorothea Dix: New England Reformer*. Cambridge, Mass.: Harvard University Press, 1998.

Burton, Brian K. *Extraordinary Circumstances: The Seven Days Battles*. Bloomington: Indiana University Press, 2001.

Calcutt, Rebecca Barbour. *Richmond's Wartime Hospitals*. Gretna, La.: Pelican Publishing, 2005.

Camp, Stephanie M. H. *Closer to Freedom: Enslaved Women and Everyday Resistance in the Plantation South*. Chapel Hill: University of North Carolina Press, 2004.

Carmichael, Peter S. *The Last Generation: Young Virginians in Peace, Warm and Reunion*. Chapel Hill: University of North Carolina Press, 2005.

Clarke, Frances M. *War Stories: Suffering and Sacrifice in the Civil War North*. Chicago: University of Chicago Press, 2011.

Cohen, Benjamin R. *Notes from the Ground: Science, Soil, and Society in the American Countryside*. New Haven, Conn.: Yale University Press, 2009.

Cowdrey, Albert E. *This Land, This South: An Environmental History*. Louisville: University Press of Kentucky, 1996.

Cozzens, Peter. *Shenandoah 1862: Stonewall Jackson's Valley Campaign*. Chapel Hill: University of North Carolina Press, 2008.

Cunningham, H. H. *Doctors in Gray: The Confederate Medical Service*. Baton Rouge: Louisiana State University Press, 1958.

Cushman, Stephen. *Bloody Promenade: Reflections on a Civil War Battle*. Charlottesville: University of Virginia Press, 1999.

Dean, Eric T. Jr. *Shook over Hell: Post-Traumatic Stress, Vietnam, and the Civil War*. Cambridge, Mass.: Harvard University Press, 1997.

Denney, Robert E. *Civil War Medicine: Care and Comfort of the Wounded*. New York: Sterling, 1994.

Dougherty, Kevin. *Civil War Leadership and Mexican War Experience*. Jackson: University Press of Mississippi, 2007.

Downer, Edward T. *Stonewall Jackson's Shenandoah Valley Campaign, 1862*. Lexington, Va.: Stonewall Jackson Memorial, 1960.

Downs, Jim. *Sick from Freedom: African-American Illness and Suffering during the Civil War and Reconstruction*. New York: Oxford University Press, 2012.

Faust, Drew Gilpin. *This Republic of Suffering: Death and the American Civil War*. New York: Alfred A. Knopf, 2008.

Fredrickson, George M. *The Inner Civil War: Northern Intellectuals and the Crisis of the Union*. 1965. Reprint, New York: Harper & Row, 1968.

Freemon, Frank R. *Gangrene and Glory: Medical Care during the American Civil War*. Madison, N.J.: Fairleigh Dickinson University Press, 1998.

Gallagher, Gary W., ed. *The Richmond Campaign of 1862: The Peninsula and the Seven Days*. Chapel Hill: University of North Carolina Press, 2000.

———. *The Shenandoah Valley Campaign of 1862*. Chapel Hill: University of North Carolina Press, 2003.

Giesberg, Judith Ann. *Civil War Sisterhood: The U.S. Sanitary Commission and Women's Politics in Transition*. Boston: Northeastern University Press, 2000.

Ginzberg, Lori D. *Women and the Work of Benevolence: Morality, Politics, and Class in the Nineteenth-Century United States*. New Haven, Conn.: Yale University Press, 1990.

Glatthaar, Joseph T. *General Lee's Army: From Victory to Collapse*. New York: Free Press, 2008.

————. *March to the Sea and Beyond: Sherman's Troops in the Savannah and Carolinas Campaigns*. Baton Rouge: Louisiana State University Press, 1995.

Green, Carol C. *Chimborazo: The Confederacy's Largest Hospital*. Knoxville: University of Tennessee Press, 2004.

Greenbie, Marjorie Barstow. *Lincoln's Daughters of Mercy*. New York: Putnam, 1944.

Haller, John S. Jr. *American Medicine in Transition 1840–1910*. Urbana: University of Illinois Press, 1981.

————. *The History of American Homeopathy: The Academic Years, 1820–1935*. Binghamton, N.Y.: Hawthorne Press, 2005.

Halliday, Stephen. *The Great Filth: The War against Disease in Victorian England*. Gloucestershire: Sutton Publishing, 2007.

Harsh, Joseph L. *Taken at the Flood: Robert E. Lee and Confederate Strategy in the Maryland Campaign of 1862*. Kent, Oh.: Kent State University Press, 1999.

Hess, Earl J. *The Union Soldier in Battle: Enduring the Ordeal of Combat*. Lawrence: University Press of Kansas, 1997.

Hume, Edgar Erskine. *Victories of Army Medicine*. Philadelphia: J. P. Lippincott, 1943.

Humphreys, Margaret. *Intensely Human: The Health of the Black Soldier in the American Civil War*. Baltimore: Johns Hopkins University Press, 2008.

Jimerson, Randall C. *The Private Civil War: Popular Thought during the Sectional Conflict*. Baton Rouge: Louisiana State University Press, 1994.

Kett, Joseph F. *The Formation of the American Medical Profession: The Roles of Institutions, 1780–1860*. New Haven, Conn.: Yale University Press, 1968.

Krick, Robert K. *Civil War Weather in Virginia*. Tuscaloosa: University of Alabama Press, 2007.

Lawson, Melinda. *Patriot Fires: Forging a New American Nationalism in the Civil War North*. Lawrence: University Press of Kansas, 2002.

Linderman, Gerald F. *Embattled Courage: The Experience of Combat in the American Civil War*. New York: Free Press, 1987.

Livermore, Thomas L. *Numbers & Losses in the American Civil War, 1861–65*. Bloomington: Indiana University Press, 1957.

Long, Everette B., with Barbara Long. *The Civil War Day by Day: An Almanac, 1861–1865*. Garden City, N.Y.: Doubleday, 1971.

Lonn, Ella. *Desertion during the Civil War*. 1928. Reprint, Lincoln: University of Nebraska Press, 1998.

Lowry, Thomas P., and Jack D. Welsh. *Tarnished Scalpels: The Court-Martials of Fifty Union Surgeons*. Mechanicsburg, Pa.: Stackpole Books, 2000.

Lystra, Karen. *Searching the Heart: Women, Men, and Romantic Love in Nineteenth-Century America*. New York: Oxford University Press, 1989.

Manning, Chandra. *What This Cruel War Was Over: Soldiers, Slavery, and the Civil War*. New York: Vintage, 2008.

Marvell, William. *Burnside*. Chapel Hill: University of North Carolina Press, 1991.

Maxwell, William Quentin. *Lincoln's Fifth Wheel*. New York: Longmans, Green, 1956.

McClurken, Jeffrey W. *Take Care of the Living: Reconstructing Confederate Veteran Families in Virginia*. Charlottesville: University of Virginia Press, 2009.

McPherson, James M. *For Cause and Comrades: Why Men Fought in the Civil War*. New York: Oxford University Press, 1997.

———. *This Mighty Scourge: Perspectives on the Civil War*. New York: Oxford University Press, 2007.

Mitchell, Reid. *Civil War Soldiers: Their Expectations and Their Experiences*. New York: Viking, 1988.

Nash, Roderick. *Wilderness and the American Mind*. 1967. Reprint, New Haven, Conn.: Yale University Press, 1982.

Nelson, Megan Kate. *Ruin Nation: Destruction and the American Civil War*. Athens: University of Georgia Press, 2012.

Numbers, Ronald L., and Todd L. Savitt, eds. *Science and Medicine in the Old South*. Baton Rouge: Louisiana State University Press, 1989.

Platt, Harold L. *Shock Cities: The Environmental Transformation and Reform of Manchester and Chicago*. Chicago: University of Chicago Press, 2005.

Rable, George C. *Civil Wars: Women and the Crisis of Southern Nationalism*. Urbana: University of Illinois Press, 1989.

———. *Fredericksburg! Fredericksburg!* Chapel Hill: University of North Carolina Press, 2002.

Robertson, James I. *The Stonewall Brigade*. Baton Rouge: Louisiana State University Press, 1978.

———. *Stonewall Jackson: The Man, the Soldier, the Legend*. New York: Macmillan, 1997.

Rogers, Naomi. *An Alternative Path: The Making and Remaking of Hahnemann Medical College and Hospital of Philadelphia*. New Brunswick, N.J.: Rutgers University Press, 1998.

Rosenberg, Charles E. *The Care of Strangers: The Rise of America's Hospital System*. New York: Basic Books, 1987.

———. *No Other Gods: On Science and American Social Thought*. Baltimore: Johns Hopkins University Press, 1961.

Rothstein, William G. *American Physicians in the Nineteenth Century: From Sects to Science*. Baltimore: Johns Hopkins University Press, 1972.

Royster, Charles. *The Destructive War: William Tecumseh Sherman, Stonewall Jackson, and the Americans*. New York: Vintage Books, 1991.

Russell, Edmund P. *War and Nature: Fighting Humans and Insects with Chemicals from World War I to Silent Spring*. Cambridge: Cambridge University Press, 2001.

Rutkow, Ira. *Bleeding Blue and Gray: Civil War Surgery and the Evolution of American Medicine*. New York: Random House, 2005.

Sears, Stephen W. *To the Gates of Richmond: The Peninsula Campaign*. New York: Ticknor & Fields, 1992.

Schantz, Mark S. *Awaiting the Heavenly Country: The Civil War and America's Culture of Death*. Ithaca, N.Y.: Cornell University Press, 2008.

Schroeder-Lein, Glenna R. *Confederate Hospitals on the Move: Samuel H. Stout and the Army of Tennessee*. Columbia: University of South Carolina Press, 1994.

———. *The Encyclopedia of Civil War Medicine*. Armonk, N.Y.: M. E. Sharpe, 2008.

Schultz, Jane E. *Women at the Front: Hospital Workers in Civil War America*. Chapel Hill: University of North Carolina Press, 2004.

Schwab, John C. *The Confederate States of America: 1861–1862: A Financial and Industrial History of the South during the Civil War*. New York: Charles Scribner's Sons, 1901.

Sheehan-Dean, Aaron, ed. *The View from the Ground: Experiences of Civil War Soldiers*. Lexington: University Press of Kentucky, 2007.

———. *Why Confederates Fought: Family and Nation in Civil War Virginia*. Chapel Hill: University of North Carolina Press, 2007.

Sicherman, Barbara. *The Quest for Mental Health in America, 1880–1917*. New York: Arno Press, 1980.

Smith, George Winston. *Medicines for the Union Army*. Madison, Wisc.: American Institute of the History of Pharmacy, 1962.

Starr, Paul. *The Social Transformation of American Medicine*. New York: Basic Books, 1984.

Steinberg, Theodore. *Down to Earth: Nature's Role in American History*. New York: Oxford University Press, 2002.

Steiner, Paul E. *Disease in the Civil War: Natural Biological Warfare in 1861–65*. Springfield, Ill.: Charles C. Thomas, 1968.

Symonds, Craig L. *Joseph E. Johnston: A Civil War Biography*. New York: W. W. Norton, 1992.

Tanner, Robert G. *Stonewall in the Valley: Thomas J. "Stonewall" Jackson's Shenandoah Valley Campaign, Spring 1862*. 1976. Reprint, Mechanicsville, Pa.: Stackpole Books, 1996.

Valencius, Conevery Bolton. *The Health of the Country: How American Settlers Understood Themselves and Their Land*. New York: Basic Books, 2002.

Warner, John Harley. *The Therapeutic Perspective: Medical Practice, Knowledge, and Identity in America, 1820–1885*. Cambridge, Mass.: Harvard University Press, 1986.

Webb, James L. A., Jr. *Humanity's Burden: A Global History of Malaria*. Cambridge: Cambridge University Press, 2009.

Weitz, Mark A. *A Higher Duty: Desertion among Georgia Troops during the War*. Lincoln: University of Nebraska Press, 2000.

———. *More Damning Than Slaughter: Desertion in the Confederate Army*. Lincoln: University of Nebraska Press, 2005.

Welsh, Jack D. *Medical Histories of Union Generals*. Kent, Oh.: Kent State University Press, 1996.

Wetherington, Mark V. *Plain Folk's Fight: The Civil War and Reconstruction in Piney Woods Georgia*. Chapel Hill: University of North Carolina Press, 2005.

Whorton, James C. *Nature Cures: The History of Alternative Medicine in America*. New York: Oxford University Press, 2002.

Wiley, Bell Irvin. *The Life of Billy Yank: The Common Soldier of the Union.* Garden City, N.Y.: Doubleday, 1952.

———. *The Life of Johnny Reb: The Common Soldier of the Confederacy.* 1943. Reprint, Baton Rouge: Louisiana State University Press, 1978.

Winders, Richard Bruce. *Mr. Polk's Army: The American Military Experience in the Mexican War.* College Station: Texas A&M University Press, 1997.

Winters, Harold A., et al., eds. *Battling the Elements: Weather and Terrain in the Conduct of War.* Baltimore: Johns Hopkins University Press, 1998.

Wyatt-Brown, Bertram. *Hearts of Darkness: Wellsprings of a Southern Literary Tradition.* Baton Rouge: Louisiana State University Press, 2003.

———. *Southern Honor: Ethics and Behavior in the Old South.* New York: Oxford University Press, 1982.

Articles and Chapters

Adams, George Worthington. "Confederate Medicine." *Journal of Southern History* 6 (May 1940): 151–66.

Black, Brian. "Addressing the Nature of Gettysburg: 'Addition and Detraction' in Preserving an American Shrine." In *Militarized Landscapes: From Gettysburg to Salisbury Plain,* ed. Chris Pearson, Peter Coates, and Tim Cole, 171–88. London: Continuum, 2010.

Bohannon, Keith. "Dirty, Ragged, and Ill-Provided For: Confederate Logistical Problems in the 1862 Maryland Campaign and Their Solutions." In *The Antietam Campaign,* ed. Gary W. Gallagher, 101–42. Chapel Hill: University of North Carolina Press, 1999.

Bollet, Alfred Jay. "The Major Infectious Epidemic Diseases of Civil War Soldiers." *Infectious Disease Clinics of North America* 18 (June 2004): 293–309.

———. "Rheumatic Diseases among Civil War Troops." *Arthritis & Rheumatism* 34 (December 2005): 1197–1203.

———. "Scurvy and Chronic Diarrhea in Civil War Troops: Were They Both Nutritional Deficiency Syndrome?" *Journal of the History of Medicine and Allied Sciences* 47 (1992): 49–67.

Bowers, Russell V. "A Confederate General Hospital: Chimborazo Post (1862–1865)." *The Scarab: Medical College of Virginia Alumni Magazine* (November 1962). http://www.mdgorman.com/Hospitals/chimborazo_hospital__bowers.htm. Accessed October 2011.

Brady, Lisa. "The Wilderness of War: Nature and Strategy." *Environmental History* 10 (July 2003): 421–77.

Braun, Lundy. "Spirometry, Measurement, and Race in the Nineteenth Century." *Journal of the History of Medicine and Allied Science* 60 (June 2005): 135–69.

Carmichael, Peter S. "So Far from God and So Close to Stonewall Jackson: The Executions of Three Shenandoah Valley Soldiers." *Virginia Magazine of History and Biography* 111 (2003): 33–66.

———. "Turner Ashby's Appeal." In *The Shenandoah Valley Campaign of 1862,* ed. Gary W. Gallagher, 144–77. Chapel Hill: University of North Carolina Press, 2003.

Cassidy, James H. "Medical Men and the Ecology of the Old South." In *Science and Medicine in the Old South*, ed. Ronald L. Numbers and Todd L. Savitt, 66–179. Baton Rouge: Louisiana State University Press, 1989.

Dean, Eric T. Jr. "Dangled over Hell: The Trauma of the Civil War." In *The Civil War Soldier: A Historical Reader*, ed. Michael Barton and Larry M. Logue, 396–421. New York: New York University Press, 2007.

Fiege, Mark. "Gettysburg and the Organic Nature of the Civil War." In *Natural Enemy, Natural Ally: Toward an Environmental History of Warfare*, ed. Richard P. Tucker and Edmund P. Russell, 93–109. Corvallis: Oregon State University Press, 2004.

Gallagher, Gary W. "You Must Either Attack Richmond or Give Up the Job and Come to the Defence of Washington: Abraham Lincoln and the 1862 Shenandoah Valley Campaign." In *The Shenandoah Valley Campaign of 1862*, ed. Gary W. Gallagher, 3–23. Chapel Hill: University of North Carolina Press, 2003.

Glatthaar, Joseph T. "Confederate Soldiers in Virginia, 1861." In *Virginia at War, 1861*, ed. William C. Davis and James I. Robertson Jr., 45–63. Lexington: University Press of Kentucky, 2005.

Grayson, Carmen Brissette. "Military Advisor to Stanton and Lincoln: Quartermaster General Montgomery C. Meigs and the Peninsula Campaign, January–August, 1862." In *The Peninsula Campaign of 1862: Yorktown to the Seven Days*, 3 vols., ed. William J. Miller, 2:73–110. Campbell, Calif.: Savas Woodbury, 1993.

Haller, John S. "Civil War Anthropometry: The Making of a Radical Ideology." *Civil War History* 16 (1970): 309–24.

Kirby, Jack Temple. "The American Civil War: An Environmental View." National Humanities Center website, *Nature Transformed: The Environment in American History* (revised July 2001). http://nationalhumanitiescenter.org/tserve/nattrans/ntuseland/essays/amcwar.htm. Accessed October 2011.

Lash, Gary G. "'No Praise Can Be Too Good for the Officers and Men': The 71st Pennsylvania Infantry in the Peninsula Campaign." In *The Peninsula Campaign of 1862: Yorktown to the Seven Days*, 3 vols., ed. William J. Miller, 3:24–59. Campbell, Calif.: Savas Woodbury, 1997.

Maslowski, Peter. "A Study of Morale in Civil War Soldiers." *Military Affairs* 34 (December 1970): 122–26.

McBride, Stephen W., and Kim A. McBride. "Civil War Housing Insights from Camp Nelson, Kentucky." In *Huts and History: The Historical Archaeology of Military Encampment during the American Civil War*, ed. Clarence R. Geier, David G. Orr, and Matthew B. Reeves, 136–72. Gainesville: University Press of Florida, 2006.

Meier, Kathryn Shively. "Fighting in 'Dante's Inferno': Changing Perceptions of Civil War Combat in the Spotsylvania Wilderness from 1863 to 1864." In *Militarized Landscapes: From Gettysburg to Salisbury Plain*, ed. Chris Pearson, Peter Coates, and Tim Cole, 39–59. London: Continuum, 2010.

———. "'This Is No Place for the Sick': Nature's War on Civil War Soldier Mental and Physical Health in the 1862 Peninsula and Shenandoah Valley Campaigns." *Journal of the Civil War Era* 1 (June 2011): 176–206.

Miller, William J. "I Wait Only for the River: McClellan and His Engineers on the Chickahominy." In *The Richmond Campaign of 1862: The Peninsula and the Seven Days*, ed. Gary Gallagher, 44–65. Chapel Hill: University of North Carolina Press, 2000.

———. "Such Men as Shields, Banks, and Frémont: Federal Command in Western Virginia, March–June 1862." In *The Shenandoah Valley Campaign of 1862*, ed. Gary W. Gallagher, 43–85. Chapel Hill: University of North Carolina Press, 2003.

Mitchell, Reid. "Not the General but the Soldier: The Study of Civil War Soldiers." In *Writing the Civil War: The Quest to Understand*, ed. James M. McPherson and William J. Cooper Jr., 81–95. Columbia: University of South Carolina Press, 2000.

Nash, Linda. "Finishing Nature: Harmonizing Bodies and Environments in Late Nineteenth-Century California." *Environmental History* 8 (January 2003): 25.

Patterson, K. David. "Disease Environments of the Antebellum South." In *Science and Medicine in the Old South*, ed. Ronald L. Numbers and Todd L. Savitt, 152–66. Baton Rouge: Louisiana State University Press, 1989.

Reiger, John F. "Deprivation, Disaffection, and Desertion in Confederate Florida Deprivation, Disaffection, and Desertion in Confederate Florida." *Florida Historical Quarterly* 48 (January 1970): 279–98.

Rosenberg, Charles E. "Medical Text and Social Context: Explaining William Buchan's Domestic Medicine." *Bulletin of the History of Medicine* 57 (1983): 22–42.

Ruffner, Kevin C. "Civil War Desertion from a Black Belt Regiment: An Examination of the 44th Virginia Infantry." In *The Edge of the South: Life in Nineteenth-Century Virginia*, ed. Edward L. Ayers and John C. Willis, 79–108. Charlottesville: University of Virginia Press, 1991.

Rutkow, Ira M. "Anesthesia during the Civil War." *Archives of Surgery* 134 (June 1999): 680.

———. "Homeopaths, Surgery, and the Civil War: Edward C. Franklin and the Struggle to Achieve Medical Pluralism in the Union Army." *Archives of Surgery* 139 (July 2004): 785–91.

Shannon, Fred A. "The Life of the Common Soldier in the Union Army, 1861–1865." In *The Civil War Soldier: A Historical Reader*, ed. Michael Barton and Larry M. Logue, 92–107. New York: New York University Press, 2007.

Stroud, Ellen. "Reflections from Six Feet under the Field: Dead Bodies in the Classroom." *Environmental History* 8 (October 2003): 618.

Taylor, Amy Murrell. "How a Cold Snap in Kentucky Led to Freedom for Thousands: An Environmental Story of Emancipation." In *Weirding the War: Stories From the Civil War's Ragged Edges*, ed. Stephen Berry, 191–214. Athens: University of Georgia Press.

Taylor, W. H. "Some Experiences of a Confederate Surgeon." In College of Physicians of Philadelphia, *Transactions*, ser. 3, vol. 28 (1906).

Warner, John Harley. "The Idea of Southern Medical Distinctiveness: Medical Knowledge and Practice in the Old South." In *Science and Medicine in the Old South*, ed. Ronald L. Numbers and Todd L. Savitt, 179–206. Baton Rouge: Louisiana State University Press, 1989.

————. "Orthodoxy and Otherness: Homeopathy and Regular Medicine in Nineteenth-Century America." In *Culture, Knowledge, and Healing: Historical Perspectives of Homeopathic Medicine in Europe and North America*, ed. Robert Jütte, Guenter B. Risse, and John Woodward, 5–29. Sheffield, U.K.: European Association for the History of Health and Medicine, 1998.

Warner, Margaret H. "Public Health in the Old South." In *Science and Medicine in the Old South*, ed. Ronald L. Numbers and Todd L. Savitt, 226–56. Baton Rouge: Louisiana State University Press, 1989.

Whitehorne, Joseph W. A. "Blueprint for Nineteenth-Century Camps: Castramentation, 1778–1865." In *Huts and History: The Historical Archaeology of Military Encampment during the American Civil War*, ed. Clarence R. Geier, David G. Orr, and Matthew B. Reeves, 28–50. Gainesville: University Press of Florida, 2006.

Index

Absenteeism, 41, 114, 126–28, 131, 133–41, 149, 182 (n. 50). *See also* Straggling

African Americans: assistance to soldiers, 14, 117, 119, 179 (n. 89); supposed resistance to disease, 19–20, 30; newspapers, 23, 31

Ague, 47, 52

Alcohol, 28, 31, 63, 71, 112, 121–22, 133, 138

Alcoholism, 27–28, 31, 63

Alexandria, 67

Allegheny Mountains, 37, 39, 41, 83

Allopathy, 30

Ambulances, 3, 52, 77–78, 82, 86, 136–37, 140, 148

American Journal of the Medical Sciences, 20

American Medical Association, 17, 28

Anemia, 19, 104

Antietam, 78

Army Corps of Engineers, 81

Army of Northern Virginia, 35, 41, 44–46, 89, 100, 118, 121, 136, 144–45, 172 (n. 77), 173 (n. 98), 181 (n. 4), 182 (n. 28), 184 (nn. 77, 93)

Army of the Potomac, 2, 7, 14, 35, 39, 41, 44–45, 48, 61, 76, 85–89, 109, 138, 160 (n. 29), 161 (n. 38), 181 (n. 4)

Army regulations, 12, 15, 37, 64, 160 (n. 29); of sanitation and supplies, 5–6, 32, 72–77, 89, 96, 148, 157 (n. 4); of straggling, 134, 137, 140, 142

Artillery, experiences of soldiers serving in, 11, 63, 103, 105, 109, 117, 129, 135, 147

Association of Army and Navy Surgeons of the Confederate States, 79

Association of Medical Superintendents of American Institutions for the Insane, 28

Asylums, 28, 33

Autopsies, 29

Banks, Maj. Gen. Nathaniel P., 38–39, 41, 64, 138, 165 (n. 13), 172 (n. 69)

Bath County, 38, 54

Bathing: as self-care, 2, 61, 73, 100–104, 172 (n. 74), 175 (n. 3), 176 (n. 6); antebellum, 32; required by officers, 32, 150. *See also* Hygiene, personal

Batholow, Dr. Robert, 150–51

Beaver Dam Creek, battle of, 44

Beds, 6, 22, 46, 54, 57, 85, 104–5, 107, 114–23 passim. *See also* Self-care: techniques: protection from elements; Sleep

Bellows, Henry Whitney, 75, 80

Benjamin, Judah P., 142–43, 164 (n. 10)

Bichat, Xavier, 29

Big Sandy, 41

Blankets, 38, 47, 56, 58, 66, 71, 89, 104–5, 109, 115, 119–20, 123, 129–31, 144

Blenker, Brig. Gen. Louis, 82, 138

Blood poisoning, 84, 93

Blue mass. *See* Mercury

Blue Ridge Mountains, 37

Boston Journal, 106

Botanico-Medical College of Ohio, 31, 150

Bowel complaints, 18, 23, 53, 59–60, 92, 96, 113, 115. *See also* Diarrhea; Dysentery

toward, 65, 74, 80, 92, 97, 141, 146, 149; surgeons' attitude toward, 92, 94; attitudes toward leave, 142–45

Commissaries, 119, 145, 173 (n. 93)

Commissary Department, 62, 65, 160 (n. 29)

Commission of Inquiry and Advice in Respect of the Sanitary interests of the United States forces. *See* Sanitary Commission, U.S.

Confederate States Medical and Surgical Journal, 79

Congress, Confederate, 135, 144

Congress, Provisional, 78

Congress, U.S., 77, 80

Conscript Act of 1862, 135

Conscription, 135–37, 182 (nn. 44, 45)

Constitutional theory of health, 8, 26, 150, 171 (n. 53)

Consumption. *See* Tuberculosis

Cooking, 5–6, 48, 77, 85–88, 91, 103–4, 108, 111, 117, 119–22, 129, 148, 150, 179 (n. 89), 180 (n. 108)

Cooper, Adj. Gen. Samuel, 137

Correspondence, 16, 49, 52–53, 57–58, 157 (n. 2); as self-care, 4, 8, 12, 14, 62–63, 69, 72, 99, 114, 117–24; as historical source, 7–8, 11, 128

Court martial, 63, 128, 137. *See also* Punishment

Cowardice, 11, 120, 126, 128, 133, 137, 141. *See also* Masculinity

Crimean War, 75, 83

Cross Keys, battle of, 41

Danville, 68, 149

Darwin, Charles, 26

Davis, Jefferson, 44–45, 79, 89, 137, 164 (n. 10)

Death: experiences with and attitudes toward, 3, 9, 15, 19–20, 22, 24, 30, 35–36, 46, 54, 56, 61, 63–64, 68, 92, 116, 120, 138, 158 (n. 9), 159 (n. 11), 169 (n. 122), 178 (n. 71); and decomposition as cause of contamination

and discomfort, 21, 52–54, 89, 105, 110–11, 134, 159 (n. 15)

Death penalty. *See* Punishment: capital

Deforestation, 1, 105, 108, 176 (n. 27). *See also* Camp: effects on environment

Dehydration, 111, 175 (n. 5). *See also* Thirst; Water

DeLeon, David C., 78

Depression, 1, 3, 7, 10, 12–13, 26, 46, 49, 54, 58–68 passim, 87, 93, 100, 106, 113, 120, 123, 131, 133, 140, 147, 150–51, 158 (nn. 9, 10), 159 (n. 11), 161 (n. 36). *See also* Mental health

Desertion, 83, 127, 128, 133–45 passim, 150, 158 (n. 6), 180 (n. 2), 181 (nn. 6, 7), 182 (nn. 28, 45), 183 (n. 62), 184 (n. 93)

Diarrhea, 6, 10, 18, 21, 25–26, 42, 45, 47–48, 53–54, 56, 59–60, 69–70, 77, 86–87, 90, 92–93, 95, 100, 111, 115, 122–23, 131, 149, 174 (n. 122), 180 (nn. 107, 108). *See also* Bowel complaints

Diet, 2, 6, 10, 12, 25–26, 28, 30–32, 53, 57, 59, 62–63, 71, 75, 81, 85–97 passim, 106, 108, 112–17, 119, 123–24, 132, 138, 147–50, 158 (n. 7), 168 (n. 118), 173 (n. 98), 180 (nn. 107, 108), 181 (n. 6). *See also* Cooking

Diphtheria, 7, 19, 35

Discipline, military, 5, 10–11, 14, 28, 33, 44–45, 63, 66, 73, 76, 88–89, 96, 106, 125–41 passim, 145, 161 (n. 38), 169 (n. 6), 183 (n. 62). *See also* Straggling

Disease: assumed causes, 3, 8, 13, 25–31, 54, 148, 150–51, 171 (n. 53), 185 (n. 7); among new recruits, 7, 13, 20, 35, 74–76, 80, 89, 124, 150. *See also names of individual diseases and vectors*

Disease environments, 4, 9, 10, 14, 19–21, 37, 58

Disinfectants, 75. *See also* Soap

Dix, Dorothea, 33

Doctors. *See* Physicians; Surgeons

physical health, 2, 12–13, 46, 54, 58, 64, 87, 93, 131, 133, 150; and self-care, 3, 7, 10, 100, 106, 113, 120, 126. *See also* Morale

Mental Hygiene, 28

Mercury: as medicine, 3, 25–26, 70, 92, 115, 163 (n. 39)

Mexican-American War, 6, 14, 74–75, 96, 157 (n. 3)

Miasma, 3, 18, 20–21, 32, 42, 52–53, 56, 59–60, 79, 82, 85, 93, 150

Migration, 17, 49

Military discipline. *See* Discipline, military

Milroy, Brig. Gen. Robert H., 39

Mobilization, 79, 148. *See also* Enlistment

Moore, Samuel Preston, 78–79, 140

Morale, 2–14 passim, 28, 32, 46, 51, 58–59, 61–63, 76, 81–82, 87–88, 104, 111, 121, 137, 144, 150, 158 (n. 9), 161 (n. 36), 184 (n. 77). *See also* Mental health; Straggling

Mortality, 46, 75, 158 (n. 9); from malaria, 19, 52; from dysentery and diarrhea, 45, 59; from battle, 52; from pneumonia, 115

Mosquitoes, 1–3, 5, 10, 18, 42, 52, 54–56, 100, 108–9, 151, 177 (n. 45), 185 (n. 7)

Mosquito nets, 71, 177 (n. 45)

Mountain Department, 39

Mount Jackson, 81

Mud, 6, 46, 47, 50–52, 87, 90, 94, 106, 108, 121, 123, 161 (n. 36); as cause of straggling, 130–31, 133, 135

Mumps, 7, 32, 35

National ERA, 23, 31

Nature: perceived relation to health in wartime, 2–16 passim, 33, 35–37, 45–64 passim, 70–71, 75–82, 86–89, 92, 94, 100, 108, 117, 119, 121, 127, 129–32, 148–51; defined, 12; perceived relation to health in antebellum period, 17–21, 28, 31–33

Navy, Confederate, 79

Navy, Union, 79, 85

Neuralgia, 69

Newspapers, 23, 31, 41, 50–51, 78, 92, 96–97, 102, 106–7, 150; health care advice in, 4, 12, 14, 19, 22–24, 117, 121–22; attitude toward common soldiers, 33, 66, 72, 95–96, 136, 138, 146; attitude to command and medical infrastructure, 65, 97. *See also* Civilians

New York Evening Post, 23

Northwest Indian wars, 82

Nostalgia, 10, 12, 61–62, 93, 150, 158 (n. 9)

Nurses, 22, 33, 66, 69, 71, 75, 77–78, 91, 94, 121; soldiers nursing each other, 113–15

Oak Grove, battle of, 44

Officers, 42, 64, 143, 157 (n. 4), 169 (n. 2); and common soldiers' health, 2–5, 7, 32–33, 37–38, 46–48, 62–66, 71–73, 76–79, 85–87, 89–90, 97, 101, 114–15, 124, 127, 133, 138, 140, 144, 146, 148, 168 (n. 110), 170 (n. 36), 173 (nn. 91, 103), 178 (n. 75); extra resources for self-care, 36, 46, 94, 100, 105–6, 112, 114, 117, 119, 133, 168 (n. 118), 177 (n. 45), 182 (n. 34); and straggling, 128–45 passim. *See also* Command

Official Records of the War of the Rebellion, The, 12

Olmsted, Frederick Law, 75–76, 80, 89–90

On Airs, Waters and Places, 18

Opium, 25–26, 92–93, 113, 163 (n. 39)

Outlines of the Chief Camp Diseases of the United States Armies, 12

Pamunkey River, 85

Parasites, 18, 57, 59, 93, 105

Pasteur, Louis, 29

Payment: wages, 103, 120, 143, 181

Straggling, 7, 10–11, 14, 60, 73, 82–83, 106, 124–50 passim, 158 (n. 6), 180 (nn. 1, 2), 181 (n. 6), 182 (n. 50), 184 (n. 93)

Strasburg, 39, 41, 64

Strong, George Templeton, 75

Stuart, Brig. Gen. J. E. B., 44

Suckley, George Cooper, 82

Suicide, 61, 63–64, 138, 158 (n. 9), 169 (n. 122)

Sunstroke, 20, 48, 59–60, 101, 121, 175 (n. 5)

Supplies. *See individual items*

Supply lines. *See* Logistics

Surgeons, 1, 3–4, 12, 27–29, 33, 50, 52, 56, 58–59, 63, 83–86, 88, 90–92, 94, 97, 137, 150, 182 (n. 42), 185 (n. 7); sickness and self-care among, 11, 62, 67, 80–81, 94–95, 106, 175 (n. 128); training and oversight of, 12, 24, 61–62, 74, 76–79, 92–93, 122, 140, 163 (n. 39), 164 (n. 10), 168 (n. 118), 172 (n. 75); soldiers' attitudes toward, 47, 66–70, 113–15, 117, 141, 169 (n. 1)

Surgery, 14, 93; emphasized over preventing illness, 15, 75, 80; accepted as treatment, 24, 162 (n. 5)

Swamps, 3, 9, 18–21, 42, 44, 48, 50–63 passim, 70, 79, 84–86, 88, 93, 105, 108, 111

Swift Run Gap, 39

Tea, 28, 71, 89

Temperance, 31

Tents, 1, 5, 6, 55, 66, 71, 73, 76, 82, 86, 88–90, 95, 104–8, 122, 138, 147; lack of, 81, 88, 92, 129, 131, 144. *See also* Exposure; Self-care: techniques: protection from elements

Thirst, 53–54, 105, 111

Thomson, Samuel, 30

Thomsonian medicine, 30–31

Ticks, 54–55, 109, 111

Trees, 1, 18, 58; as shelter, 1–2, 44, 48, 101, 105–7, 130, 133; as medicine, 25, 108, 163 (n. 39)

Tripler, Charles H., 78, 85–86, 91, 138, 141, 173 (nn. 90, 91)

Tuberculosis, 18–19, 35, 59

Typhoid, 4, 10, 18–19, 29, 42, 47, 53–54, 56, 61, 67–68, 83–86, 90, 93, 110–11, 114, 128, 131, 149

Typhus, 54, 86, 93, 95

Uniforms. *See* Clothing

U.S. Medical Bureau, 70

U.S. Sanitary Commission. *See* Sanitary Commission, U.S.

Valley Spirit, 96–97

Vector-borne disease theory, 3, 54, 148, 151, 185 (n. 7) *See also* Disease: assumed causes

Veterans. *See* Soldiers: veteran

Volunteers. *See* Soldiers: volunteer

Wages. *See* Payment

Washington, D.C., 9, 39, 72, 76–77, 80, 82, 84, 140

Water, 49, 64, 75, 85–87; contaminated, 1, 3, 5, 19, 29, 32, 35, 45, 49, 53–54, 56, 61, 73, 83, 105, 111–12, 115, 149, 180 (n. 108); obtaining for drinking, 2–3, 5, 16, 54, 58–59, 72, 84, 86, 105, 108, 111–12, 121–22, 127, 129, 132, 146–48, 158 (n. 4), 177 (n. 57), 178 (n. 84), 179 (n. 89); drainage to improve health and comfort, 3, 5, 20, 52, 79, 100, 108 (*see also* Sanitation); as element of exposure, 12, 31, 37–38, 42, 44–47, 50–53, 56, 58, 63, 70, 81, 84–87, 90, 94–95, 100, 103–6, 108, 115, 121, 123–24, 128–31, 133, 139, 147, 161 (n. 36); as medicine, 21, 30, 31; flooding, 42, 44, 84, 50, 73, 124; for bathing and laundry, 101–2, 111

Water Cure Journal, 23

Watson, Peter H., 82, 145

Weather: soldiers' preoccupation with, 2, 8, 16; perceived influence on health,

2, 10, 12, 17–21, 37, 39–42, 45–48, 50–60 passim, 64, 70–71, 81–84, 86–87, 100, 103, 106, 108, 111, 118, 121, 123–24, 134–36, 143–44, 147, 160 (n. 25), 181 (n. 6); and straggling, 129, 131, 135, 143. *See also individual aspects of weather*

Wells. *See* Water: obtaining for drinking

Western Journal of Medicine, 20

Whiskey. *See* Alcohol

White House Landing, 71, 85

White Oak Swamp, 44, 48, 56, 63; battle of, 44

Whooping cough, 7, 35

Williamsburg, 44, 64, 133,

Winchester, 38, 41, 50, 144, 164 (n. 10);

battle of, 41

Winder, Brig. Gen. Charles S., 136–37

Women, as care providers, 1, 14, 22, 31–33, 49, 67, 74–75, 78–79, 102–4, 117–19, 159 (n. 16), 162 (n. 25), 170 (n. 34), 179 (n. 94). *See also* Civilians

Women's Central Association of Relief (WCAR), 75

Woodward, Joseph Janvier, 12

Yellow fever, 18–19, 32, 52

York River, 42

Yorktown, 52, 54, 58, 85, 90, 92, 107, 112, 119; siege of, 42, 45

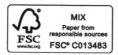